Working with Swallowing Disorders

A Multidisciplinary Approach

Jill C. Thresher, M.A., CCC-SLP

Ellis A. Kehoe, M.Ed., OTR/L

Communication Skill Builders

3830 E. Bellevue/P.O. Box 42050
Tucson, Arizona 85733
(602) 323-7500

Reproducing Pages from This Book

Many of the pages in this book can be reproduced for instructional or administrative use (not for resale). To protect your book, make a photocopy of each reproducible page. Then use that copy as a master for photocopying or other types of reproduction.

Acknowledgments

Many thanks to:

Carolyn Folds, R.D., and Andrea Groon, R.D., Hillhaven regional dietary consultants, and Judith Hirsch, dietary services manager, Hillhaven of Chapel Hill, North Carolina, for their assistance with the Dysphagia Diet, Guidelines for Determining Oral vs. Nonoral Feeding, Nutritional Assessment, and Practical Hints for Home Preparation of Food for the Adult with Dysphagia.

Frank Hielema, Ph.D., PT, Hillhaven regional associate director of rehabilitation, for his editorial assistance.

Mark Bergner, R.N., Hillhaven of Chapel Hill, North Carolina, for editorial assistance with the nursing portions of this manual.

Anne L. Gill, M.A., CCC-SLP, speech-language pathologist with University of North Carolina Hospitals, Chapel Hill, North Carolina, for editorial assistance and for the original concept of the bedside feeding and swallowing instructions sheet labeled *ATTENTION!* in Chapter 7 of this manual.

Kathy Fuller, administrative assistant, Hillhaven Corporate Office, and Nancy Dede Banks, rehabilitation department secretary at Hillhaven of Chapel Hill, for forms and manuscript preparation.

About the Authors

Jill C. Thresher, M.A., CCC-SLP, is director of speech pathology at Hillhaven Rehabilitation and Convalescent Center of Durham, North Carolina. Her responsibilities include performing diagnostic evaluations, developing treatment plans, coordinating interdisciplinary activities, scheduling, and conducting dysphagia evaluations and treatment. She also serves as a clinical practicum supervisor for graduate students from the Division of Speech and Hearing Sciences at the University of North Carolina in Chapel Hill.

Ms. Thresher received an M.A. degree in communication disorders from the University of Massachusetts. She also received a B.A. degree in speech pathology and audiology from the University of Florida.

Ellis A. Kehoe, M.Ed, OTR/L, is an employee of Communi-Care Pro-Rehab, working as the occupational therapy coordinator at Integrated Health Services at Crabtree Valley in Raleigh, North Carolina. She is also a contractor with Home Health Agency of Chapel Hill, North Carolina. In a previous position she was the director of occupational therapy at Hillhaven Convalescent Center of Chapel Hill, North Carolina. She has also served as a guest lecturer at the School of Medicine of the University of North Carolina.

Ms. Kehoe received an M.Ed. degree in elementary education, with emphasis on learning disabilities, from Tufts University Graduate School of Arts and Sciences. From the Boston School of Occupational Therapy of Tufts University she received a B.S. degree in occupational therapy. She also received an A.A. degree in liberal arts from Bradford Junior College.

Contents

1 ■ The Multidisciplinary Approach to Swallowing Disorders

Introduction

Rationale and Purpose

This manual is a guide for establishing and managing a multidisciplinary team dedicated to improving the safety, efficiency, and adequacy of oral intake in individuals with swallowing disorders, or *dysphagia*. The critical need for a concerted effort in addressing the complex needs of patients with dysphagia is underscored by the threat of aspiration pneumonia. Rehabilitative management of dysphagia, the focus of this manual, has been shown to be highly effective in reducing the incidence of aspiration pneumonia (Kasprisin et al. 1989).

A multidisciplinary approach to the coordination of patient care is a common theme in medical practice (Bach et al. 1989). This multifaceted approach is particularly applicable when traditional boundaries among professional disciplines are crossed, or when coordination of several services or therapies is indicated. Swallowing disorders are prime examples of medical conditions in which an integrated, team-based approach can be most beneficial to the patient (Bach et al. 1989).

Many patients with dysphagia have speech-production disorders (Groher 1984, p. 240). The **speech-language pathologist,** with skills in swallowing facilitation and stimulation, laryngeal functioning treatment, and oral-motor re-education and strengthening, is a key member of the multidisciplinary team.

Dysphagia rehabilitation requires the services of an **occupational therapist** for training the patient in using adaptive feeding techniques and specialized feeding equipment. In collaboration with the physical therapist, the occupational therapist also provides treatments for muscle spasticity, muscle strengthening, and eye-hand coordination, as well as for the reduction or elimination of abnormal reflexes that can interfere with feeding and swallowing (Groher 1984, p. 239).

The activities of the **nursing staff** are absolutely vital to the success of a multidisciplinary swallowing team. Often, nurses are the first to identify a patient with swallowing difficulties. Nurses are responsible for the daily monitoring of nutritional and medical status and for administering non-oral feedings. The nursing staff also ensures that aspiration precautions are maintained and provides mealtime assistance, if needed.

The **registered dietitian** must be involved to ensure that appropriate and adequate nutrition is provided, and to implement specialized dysphagia diet orders as needed.

Among the other therapists who may be involved in the management of the patient with dysphagia are the **physical therapist** and **respiratory therapist.** Patients with respiratory diseases, movement disorders, poor body positioning, or pain that interferes with the act of eating may be treated by a physical therapist. The respiratory therapist is usually not directly involved on the swallowing team, but provides valuable information regarding patients with respiratory disorders and tracheostomy tubes (Groher 1984, p. 242).

The **attending physician** often refers patients for dysphagia evaluation and rehabilitation and acts as central coordinator of the patient's medical treatment. The patient's attending physician plays a leading role in determining the best method of feeding (oral or non-oral) and makes referrals to other physician specialists.

Specialists in **otolaryngology/head and neck surgery, radiology, gastro-enterology** and **neurology** are often involved in the care of the patient with dysphagia (Miller and Groher 1990). The otolaryngologist/head and neck surgeon performs additional medical evaluation and surgical procedures for many patients with swallowing difficulties, such as those with problems involving vocal-fold approximation. Also, since disorders of the head and neck (often related to cancer) can compromise the swallowing mechanism, the otolaryngologist/head and neck surgeon frequently refers patients to the multidisciplinary team before and after corrective surgery (Miller and Groher 1990).

The radiologist works closely with the speech-language pathologist in the radiographic evaluation of the swallowing mechanism. Some referrals to the multidisciplinary team originate from the gastroenterologist, who evaluates the esophagus and lower gastrointestinal tract. Many referrals come from the neurologist, who differentially diagnoses neurological disorders. A large number of patients with disorders of neurological origin evidence swallowing difficulties.

The cooperation and involvement of **family members, friends,** and **volunteers** can be invaluable in the success of the swallowing rehabilitation program. They can provide support, follow-through, and feeding assistance (if recommended) during the hospital stay. They can also be trained by team members prior to the patient's discharge to ensure that the team recommendations will be followed for safe and adequate nutritional intake.

A number of models for multidisciplinary swallowing teams have been outlined recently (Erlichman 1989; Glickstein et al. 1989; Newman and Medina 1987; Langley 1987; Groher 1984; Logemann 1983; Steefel 1981). The establishment in 1980 of The Swallowing Center at the Johns Hopkins Hospital in

Baltimore, Maryland, serves as an example of a model, and indicates the need for a multidimensional approach to the diagnosis, treatment, and management of patients with dysphagia in medical settings. A common theme among all models is the importance of maintaining safety and adequate nutrition, ongoing training and education, and open communication and cooperation among team members, staff, and family.

The success of specific team management programs has been described in the literature. Griffin (1974) found that 15 of 17 patients placed in a multidisciplinary swallowing program successfully completed the program, eating semisolid or solid foods, and consuming liquids without choking, aspirating, or exhibiting other swallowing difficulties.

Emick-Herring and Wood (1990) reported a success rate of more than 90 percent (indicated by at least partial oral eating and drinking) for patients in a model dysphagia program that combined healthcare professionals from speech-language pathology, occupational therapy, nursing, medicine, and dietary disciplines, and incorporated individual and group dysphagia treatments. They further reported on the positive impact of this program on patient and staff satisfaction and on how the program stimulated nursing interest and confidence in the management of dysphagia.

Bach et al. (1989) described an integrated team approach with a major focus on determining the need for dietary adjustments in maintaining or restoring the safety of oral feeding in patients with dysphagia. This was accomplished through detailed radiographic examinations, development of specialized dysphagia diets, and regular evaluations by an occupational therapist, physiotherapist, and speech-language pathologist. While it was difficult to prove that this multidisciplinary team approach to dysphagia directly resulted in a decrease in aspiration and subsequent pulmonary complications, patient care was significantly improved by the comprehensive assessment and management strategies aimed at decreasing these risks.

In summary, an integrated, multidisciplinary team approach for the assessment and management of the individual with dysphagia should include the services of a speech-language pathologist, occupational therapist, registered nurse, registered dietitian, attending physician, the patient and family members, and the supportive or consultative services of additional physicians and therapists. The focus of this manual is providing a means to establish, coordinate, and evaluate the success of a multidisciplinary swallowing team in a medical setting.

Description

Working with Swallowing Disorders: A Multidisciplinary Approach will direct the medical facility's team in the successful identification and rehabilitation of adults with swallowing disorders from the moment they are admitted or identified in the facility until they have achieved safe, adequate nutritional intake. This comprehensive manual provides step-by-step guidelines throughout the stages of management, including:

- referral
- screening
- assessment
- treatment
- discharge.

Features of the manual include:

- a detailed management protocol
- inservice education suggestions
- reproducible team assessment forms with complete instructions
- a dysphagia diet
- guidelines for producing the appropriate consistency of diet items
- guidelines for determining the best feeding method.

Also included is a series of reproducible handouts and chart inserts designed to educate staff and family and to facilitate safe, efficient, adequate oral intake. The manual also provides speech-language pathology and occupational therapy treatment suggestions from which individually tailored therapy programs can be developed.

Instructional Audience

This manual was developed for use with adults who have feeding and swallowing disorders and are being cared for in medical settings (such as hospitals, subacute care facilities, rehabilitation centers, and extended care facilities) and at home.

It is designed to be used primarily with patients who have acquired neurogenic oral-pharyngeal dysphagia as a result of stroke, head injury, or progressive neurological diseases, such as multiple sclerosis or Parkinson's disease.

Some of the information in the manual can also be used in the management of mechanical swallowing disorders resulting from structural lesions, such as those that occur following treatment for cancer of the head or neck.

Swallowing disorders of esophageal origin, which are most often managed medically or surgically (rather than through rehabilitation) are beyond the scope of this manual.

Etiology of Swallowing Disorders

Swallowing disorders can result from many of the degenerative neurological diseases, as well as from stroke, head injury, or cancer of the head and neck (Erlichman 1989; Kirschner 1989; Groher 1984; Logemann 1983). Often the swallowing difficulty is the first symptom of disease (Erlichman 1989). Dysphagia can also be a result of esophageal disease arising from a motoric or structural impairment (Miller and Groher 1990; Erlichman 1989).

Swallowing function disorders are divided into three phases: oral preparatory, oropharyngeal, and esophageal (Emick-Herring and Wood 1990; Kirschner 1989; Logemann 1983; Steefel 1981; Schultz et al. 1979). From these phases, two primary types of dysphagia arise (Erlichman 1989; Castell and Donner 1987). **Oropharyngeal dysphagia** involves difficulty with oral transit and with moving food or liquid from the oral cavity through the oral pharynx into the esophagus. Patients with neuromuscular diseases account for approximately 80 percent of oropharyngeal dysphagic disorders (Erlichman 1989). **Esophageal dysphagia** involves difficulty in passing food or liquid from the esophagus to the stomach (Erlichman 1989).

Stroke (also called *cerebrovascular accident,* or *CVA*), is a prevalent cause of neuromuscular disease. The most common dysphagic symptom in stroke patients is the absence or delay in the triggering of the swallowing reflex (Logemann 1983). Patients with CVA may also exhibit paralysis of one or more structures in the vocal tract with subsequent impairments in functioning, such as loss of bolus control or oral transit difficulties secondary to lingual hemiparesis.

In the pharyngeal phase of the swallow, ingested material may fall over the base of the tongue and into the valleculae.* The material may stay there for a few seconds, until a swallow is triggered, or it may spill into the airway where it could be aspirated before the swallow reflex is triggered (Logemann 1983, p. 77). Food residue may remain in the valleculae or may collect in the pyriform sinuses* until it overflows into the trachea—again causing aspiration (Logemann 1983, p. 79).

In brainstem strokes, cricopharyngeal dysfunction is more common and involves impairment of the cricopharyngeal muscle juncture at the top of the esophagus (Groher 1984; Logemann 1983). In closed-head-injured patients, dysphagic disturbances closely parallel those found in stroke patients (Logemann 1983).

Many of the progressive neurological diseases that cause dysphagia are characterized by swallowing impairments that progress over time (Kirschner 1989; Groher 1984; Logemann 1983). Thus, frequent reevaluation of a patient's swallowing status is an important part of patient care among these individuals.

Patients with **Parkinson's disease** often show difficulty in bolus formation, tremor of the tongue or velum (Kirschner 1989), disturbed pharyngeal motility (Lieberman et al. 1980), and excessive time for oral mastication (Groher 1984, p. 130). Generally, the progression of swallowing impairment in Parkinson's disease begins with reduction in pharyngeal peristalsis and repetitive rocking motion of the tongue (Logemann 1983, p. 219). Reduction in pharyngeal peristalsis may worsen over time, laryngeal closure may become inadequate, the swallow reflex may become delayed, and cricopharyngeal dysfunction can occur (Logemann 1983, p. 210).

Patients with **amyotrophic lateral sclerosis** may have difficulty with lingual mobility, laryngeal functioning, pharyngeal peristalsis reductions, and delayed swallowing reflex (Logemann 1983, pp. 219-220). Also, these patients may evince chewing fatigue and palatal and pharyngeal weakness (Groher 1984).

Individuals with **multiple sclerosis** exhibit a variety of swallowing disorders, depending upon lesion location and cranial nerves affected (Logemann 1983, p. 220). Reduction in pharyngeal peristalsis and delay in swallowing reflex can occur with these patients (Logemann 1983, p. 220).

Myasthenia gravis can present with swallowing function which worsens with use but recovers with rest (Logemann 1983, p. 221). Mastication and swallowing may be normal at first but can deteriorate to the point where the patient is unable to chew or swallow (Groher 1984, p. 125). Some of these individuals have difficulty holding a bolus of food on the tongue (Groher 1984, p. 125-126).

NOTE: The * following words throughout the text indicates these words are found in the glossary (pages 95-97).

Typically, patients with swallowing disorders as a result of **degenerative neurologic diseases** do not show gains in swallowing functioning. They can, however, be helped to swallow more safely through positioning and modifications in diet and feeding.

Mechanical swallowing disorders can result from **acute inflammatory processes** that injure oropharyngeal tissue, such as chemical irritants or viral agents (Groher 1984, p. 61). Mechanical dysphagia can also result from **structural lesions** such as those that occur after treatment for laryngeal, oral, or oropharyngeal cancer. Dysfunctions which become apparent depend on the nature of the sensory loss (Groher 1984) and on the nature and extent of surgical treatment, resectioning, reconstructing, or radiation (Groher 1984). Esophageal dysphagia may result from **mechanical or obstructive disorders** such as peptic strictures, tumors, or webs, or from motor disorders such as achalasia* (Marshall 1985).

Some changes in swallowing functioning can occur with **advanced age.** Specifically, an increased number of chewing strokes and slower food manipulation have been noted. Adults in their 80s may experience some reduction in strength of pharyngeal and esophageal peristalsis (Feldman et al. 1980).

Considerations in Establishing a Multidisciplinary Swallowing Team

Groher (1984, p. 237) identifies a number of important considerations in establishing a multidisciplinary swallowing team. The considerations include:

- size and type of patient population
- staff attitudes towards rehabilitative management
- personnel availability
- opportunity for program development
- individual interests in dysphagia.

Goals of the Multidisciplinary Swallowing Team

Goals of the multidisciplinary swallowing team are:

- to identify patients with swallowing and chewing disorders
- to prevent aspiration and thereby to reduce the incidence of aspiration pneumonia
- to prevent malnutrition and dehydration
- to help the patient achieve safety, adequacy, and independence in swallowing, chewing, and overall oral feeding in the medical setting
- to educate staff, family, and patient about the nature and management of swallowing disorders.

Referrals

Referrals to the team may include any patient:

- on aspiration precautions or with a history of aspiration or aspiration pneumonia
- consistently exhibiting signs or symptoms of aspiration such as coughing, strangling, choking, or sneezing while eating or drinking
- suspected of having difficulty swallowing foods or liquids by mouth
- who has chewing difficulties, drooling, or copious secretions
- experiencing difficulty with swallowing medications
- being fed by tube who has, or may have, the potential for progressing to oral intake
- who is experiencing oral or nasal regurgitation.

Protocol

The following protocol describes the transition of the patient through the course of dysphagia management and the roles of the various team members at each step of management. This protocol was designed to be used in any medical setting; it can also serve as a guide to developing an individually tailored protocol to meet the needs of your specific medical setting.

1. Physician or nurse identifies patient with potential swallowing and feeding problems. This is usually done during assessment. It might also be done during admission, the patient's first meal, or when medication is administered. The nurse completes a swallowing screening form as part of the initial nursing assessment (see Chapter 3). If the patient fails the screening, the nurse obtains a physician's order for speech-language pathology and occupational therapy consults, or the physician may directly initiate referrals.

2. Speech-language pathology and occupational therapy review chart and assess patient within 24 hours. Dietitian assesses patient within 24 hours.

3. Immediate modifications as determined by assessments are implemented, such as diet modification or NPO* status.

4. If the patient is determined to be a candidate for radiographic assessments (such as videofluoroscopic swallowing or scintigraphic studies), or for additional assessments by physician specialists, these are scheduled and administered (Bass 1988; Fleming et al. 1989).

5. Team meets at rounds to review patient status, swallowing study and other assessment results, and to develop treatment plan. Team completes and posts applicable patient care information sheets, bedside feeding and swallowing instructions, NPO sheet, dysphagia flow sheet, medicine administration sheet, and aspiration precautions sheet. (These reproducible forms are located in Chapter 7.)

6. Physician orders feeding method, diet, and therapy. (Sample orders include: *advance diet as tolerated according to team recommendations* and *lunch only with occupational therapy, dysphagia puree diet.*) Tube feeding orders, if appropriate, are adjusted for those patients receiving both oral and non-oral feeding.

7. Family members are invited to scheduled team meeting when possible. Individual team members discuss treatment plan with patient and patient's family on an ongoing basis.

8. Treatment is initiated according to the roles and responsibilities of each member. Speech-language pathologist and occupational therapist may initiate trial oral feeding, if indicated. Physical therapist and respiratory therapist initiate treatment if indicated. (See Selected Feeding Management Strategies, p. 9).

9. Team meets at least weekly at rounds to monitor progress, to recommend modifications in feeding methods and facilitating strategies, and to recommend diet changes. Aspiration precautions sheets and ATTENTION! sheets are updated. Flow sheets are reviewed. Informal consults among team members are ongoing.

10. If change in diet consistency is recommended, the dietary department is notified and makes the change within two meals. If additional physician's order is necessary (such as to discontinue tube feeding), registered nurse should obtain order within 24 hours.

11. The patient is discontinued from the program once he or she achieves safe, adequate nutritional intake and maximum level of independence possible. For many patients this will be a mechanical soft diet. Physician orders discontinuation from team program.

   Often the patient is discharged from the medical facility prior to being discontinued from the program. In this case, follow-up and consultation are imperative to ease the transition from the medical setting to the home or other environment. The social worker can serve as a resource person and assist in discharge planning.

12. Quality Assurance form is completed at the team rounds at the time of the patient's discharge from the team program or the medical facility.

13. In rehabilitation or extended care medical settings, the patient may be referred to a restorative feeding program or small supervised-group feeding program following discharge from the swallowing program. In some cases, the patient may continue with the swallowing team program during the first two weeks of restorative feeding or supervised feeding group, particularly if diet modifications are still being made. See *Supervised Feeding Groups* (Appendix E, page 111) for suggested types of supervised feeding groups.

14. Registered nurse or rehabilitation nurse continues to monitor patient's swallowing, feeding, and nutritional status after discontinuation from the team program.

Selected Feeding Management Strategies

After the patient is assessed by the multidisciplinary swallowing team, one of a number of feeding-management strategies may be indicated. The strategies (adapted from Langley 1987, p. 45) include:

- Initiate or continue oral feeding as the sole means of nutritional intake. Initiate treatment, direct and indirect. Patients who have difficulty primarily with the oral phase of swallowing may be appropriate candidates for this strategy.

- Initiate oral feeding with the non-oral feeding method still in place, gradually increasing reliance on oral intake. Patients who have an impairment in swallowing, sufficient to interfere with adequate oral intake, may be considered for this strategy.

- Initiate indirect treatment with a plan of introducing oral feeding at a later date when the patient is more able. Patients who are currently unable to swallow safely or adequately but whose medical disability is expected to improve may be considered for this type of management.

- Postpone rehabilitative intervention and reassess the patient after a further period of recovery. Patients who are too ill or confused to effectively participate in a swallowing rehabilitation program, and whose potential for recovery is uncertain, should be considered for this strategy.

- Discuss the provision of a permanent alternative or aid to oral feeding. Patients who have no means of safe swallowing or for obtaining adequate oral intake, and who have a guarded prognosis for improvement, might be selected for this type of management. In some cases, surgery or prosthetic devices may offer the possibility of resuming oral feeding. In other situations, non-oral feeding methods, such as a percutaneous endoscopic gastrostomy feeding tube (PEG) must be considered.

Roles and Responsibilities of Team Members

Speech-language pathologist

Assesses oral-motor function and swallowing status. Recommends, assists, and interprets results of videofluoroscopic studies when indicated. Develops and manages exercises when indicated. Determines with physician and dietitian most appropriate feeding method (oral vs. non-oral). Recommends diet consistency and degree of supervision required. Trains patient, staff, and family in compensatory swallowing techniques. Performs ongoing determination of swallowing status. Assesses influence of language comprehension, ability to follow instructions, mental status, and overall responsiveness on swallowing. Recommends aspiration precautions as indicated.

Occupational therapist

Assesses hand-to-mouth and grasp/release patterns necessary for feeding. Determines adaptive-equipment needs and functional arm positioning to facilitate feeding independence. Assesses sensory-perceptual-motor and cognitive status as it influences feeding. Teaches patient compensatory techniques for sensory-perceptual-motor deficits as these deficits influence feeding. Assesses body positioning and physical endurance during feeding. Facilitates best body positioning for oral feeding and helps establish a functional eating time limit. Promotes cognitive and socialization skills to assist the patient in returning to a more social eating situation. Teaches staff and family techniques to facilitate functional oral feeding while using appropriate hand-to-mouth patterns. Trains staff and family in adaptive equipment use and proper body positioning methods.

Registered nurse

Identifies patients with chewing and swallowing problems upon admission, during their first meal, or when administering oral medication. Requests appropriate orders from physician and notifies team members of physician's orders. Administers and supervises oral and non-oral feedings. Monitors oral and non-oral intake and monitors patient's weight weekly or as ordered. Requests appropriate equipment to assure a safe environment (such as suction machine). Monitors patient's chewing and swallowing skills after discharge from active treatment. Ensures that all medications are appropriate for recommended food consistency. Together with the dietitian, evaluates patient's nutritional status on an ongoing basis to ensure the patient is receiving adequate intake to maintain nutrition and hydration. Rehabilitation nurses are often key team members in the ongoing management of the patient with dysphagia.

Registered dietitian

Assesses nutritional needs, adequacy of nutrient intake, and food preferences and tolerances. Screens for history of weight loss or aspiration pneumonia. Ensures that proper consistencies, temperatures, and food choices are selected for each patient, and that adequate nutrition is provided to the patient during the dysphagia rehabilitation program. This may involve recommendations regarding maintenance of non-oral feeding, or use of nutritional supplements. Obtains and reports previous dietary habits. Monitors daily nutritional intake. Does calorie counts twice weekly and monitors weight weekly. Works with speech-language pathologist and physician to determine most appropriate feeding method (oral vs. non-oral) and diet consistency.

Attending physician

Provides written orders for evaluation and treatment by team. Orders videofluoroscopic swallowing studies as indicated. Modifies orders as needed after consultation with team members. Plays leading role in decision making regarding oral/non-oral feeding procedures and medical management procedures. Provides reinforcement of swallowing procedures with patients.

Physician specialists

Otolaryngologist/head and neck surgeon. Refers patients pre- and post-operatively for cancer of the oropharyngeal or laryngeal areas. Performs direct or indirect laryngoscopy to examine for vocal fold approximation, lesions, and degree of laryngeal excursion during swallowing. Performs related surgical procedures (such as removal of vocal fold lesions, administration of therapeutic injections for airway protection, cricopharyngeal myotomy,* or procedures to control excessive saliva [Miller and Groher 1990, p. 28]).

Radiologist. Administers and interprets radiographic studies (such as the videofluoroscopic swallowing study) with the speech-language pathologist.

Gastroenterologist. Diagnoses and treats diseases that involve the esophagus and gastrointestinal tract. Refers patients for additional swallowing evaluation.

Neurologist. Examines cranial nerves involved in the swallowing process. Refers patients post-stroke or neurological injury. Differentially diagnoses and manages patients manifesting neurological disorders.

Other therapists

Physical therapist. Assesses movement and posture. Treats patients with respiratory disease—often in conjunction with respiratory therapist. Respiratory treatment may include deep suction and postural drainage (Langley 1987, p. 9). Works with occupational therapist in suppression of abnormal reflexes, pain management during feeding, and determination of appropriate body positioning and devices.

Respiratory therapist. Assesses and monitors pulmonary status. Makes recommendations for removal of tracheostomy tubes, provides consultation on choice of tracheostomy tube and how the tube is to be used in feeding (Groher 1984, p. 242). Aids in the management of oxygen use and in other respiratory treatment techniques.

Family

Attends weekly team meetings. Assists with mealtime management if recommended by team. Provides patient with support and followthrough during rehabilitation.

2 ■ Inservice Education

Introduction

Three areas of inservice education are recommended when establishing a multidisciplinary swallowing team. The **first** area is the education of the team members, which includes the speech-language pathologist, the occupational therapist, the registered nurse, the registered dietitian, and other therapists, if indicated.

The **second** area is the education of professionals not directly involved with the daily implementation of the multidisciplinary swallowing program, such as physicians, administrators, and consultants.

The **third** area is the training and management of professionals/paraprofessionals directly involved in the ongoing implementation of the multidisciplinary swallowing program. Included here are licensed practical nurses, nursing assistants and rehabilitation assistants, and dietary personnel.

A variety of training methods can be used, such as lectures, demonstrations, audiovisual aids, self-correcting quizzes, and videotape showings of dysphagia training tapes (for a list of training videos, see Appendix F, page 112). A week of highlighting team responsibilities and activities can be held annually. Additionally, all newly hired staff should be provided with inservice education during the initial orientation period.

Educating Team Members

The team members will educate one another during the initial weekly multidisciplinary swallowing team rounds and on an as-needed basis.

Objectives

The objectives for inservice education are for each team member to:

- become familiar with each member's role and responsibility on the team

- become familiar with each member's perception of the patient with respect to swallowing, chewing, and oral feeding

- have an understanding of the basic assessments, specialized assessment techniques, various adaptive equipment, and proper body positioning for oral feeding

- be familiar with the various forms being used by the team and be able to explain their use to staff and family.

Guidelines

Various members of the multidisciplinary swallowing team can give valuable inservice presentations. The **speech-language pathologist** can talk about:

- etiology of swallowing disorders

- prognosis

- clinical signs and symptoms of aspiration

- swallowing evaluation

- dysphagia severity levels

- videofluoroscopic swallowing studies—criteria, rationale, results, and implications.

The **occupational therapist** can give presentations relating to:

- adaptive equipment

- positioning techniques

- feeding evaluation

- physical and verbal feeding assistance.

The **registered nurse** can discuss:

- the swallowing screening form

- tube-feeding

- aspiration precautions

- administering medications

- suctioning

- oral hygiene.

The **registered dietitian** can talk about:

- determining the percentage of food consumed

- dysphagia diets

- adequacy of intake

- dietary assessments.

Physicians, Administrators, and Consultants

The education of physicians, administrators, and consultants is vital to the success of the multidisciplinary swallowing team program.

Objectives

The objectives for educating these individuals are to:

- present the goals and benefits of the multidisciplinary swallowing program
- help them become familiar with this manual
- summarize the roles and responsibilities of each team member
- discuss criteria used to make a referral to the program
- identify various patients targeted for this program.

Guidelines

Suggested guidelines for educating physicians, administrators, and consultants include:

- encourage attendance at multidisciplinary swallowing team rounds
- circulate and review this manual
- ask team members to describe their individual roles and responsibilities
- ask team members to make mini-presentations at utilization review or other medical review committee meetings
- send a letter or brochure describing the multidisciplinary swallowing team program to area physicians.

Professional and Paraprofessional Staff

The professional and paraprofessional staff members directly involved in the implementation of the multidisciplinary swallowing program are nurses, certified nursing assistants, certified occupational therapy assistants, rehabilitation technicians, cooks, and dietary aides.

Objectives

The objectives for inservice education for professional and paraprofessional staff members are to help them learn to:

- use the Swallowing Screening Form to identify possible swallowing problems (see Chapter 3, pages 21, 43)
- recognize signs and symptoms of aspiration
- know aspiration precautions (see Chapter 7, pages 88, 94)

- know how to see and feel for the swallow (see Appendix D, page 110)

- recognize swallowing difficulties at mealtime and be able to document them on the Dysphagia Flow Sheet

- position the patient correctly for feeding

- recognize and ensure that the patient's food tray has the recommended diet consistency as indicated on the ATTENTION! sheet

- assist the patient in the use of facilitative swallowing techniques as designated on the ATTENTION! sheet

- provide necessary verbal and physical assistance during meals

- understand the Medicine Administration sheet, the ATTENTION! feeding and swallowing instructions sheet, the Dysphagia Flow Sheet, the Aspiration Precautions Sheet and the "NPO" sheet (see Chapter 7)

- determine percentage of food on a tray and volume of liquid consumed

- accurately document the amount of time it takes the patient to consume each meal.

Guidelines

Educational opportunities for professional and paraprofessional personnel include:

- designating a Multidisciplinary Swallowing Team Program week, during which team activities and responsibilities are highlighted and inservices are given by team members

- holding scheduled viewings of dysphagia training tapes with at least one member of the team present to answer questions and provide information

- asking team members, individually and as part of the group, to provide specific inservices pertaining to their areas of expertise

- asking team members to work one-on-one with individual staff members during meals with the patient (following completion of individual speech-language pathology or occupational therapy mealtime management).

Multidisciplinary Swallowing Program

Inservice Quiz

1. What is dysphagia?

2. List 3 signs/symptoms of potential swallowing problems.

   -
   -
   -

3. List 3 "bad" foods for a patient with dysphagia.

   -
   -
   -

4. What is the *Toothette®* for?

5. Into which side of the patient's mouth should you put food?

6. After putting food in the patient's mouth, how can you determine if the patient has swallowed?

7. What patient behaviors during feeding would tell you to stop feeding the patient?

8. What are aspiration precautions?

9. When and why should you use a "nosey cut-out cup?"

10. When is it safe for a certified nursing assistant to feed a patient who has been receiving swallowing training from an occupational therapist and a speech-language pathologist?

11. List 4 important facts given about the patient on the ATTENTION! sheet.

    -
    -
    -
    -

12. Who is responsible for filling out the Dysphagia Flow Sheet?

13. When should the Dysphagia Flow Sheet be completed?

14. What does the term *consistency not tolerated* refer to on the Dysphagia Flow Sheet?

15. How are "Food%" and "cc" intake determined?

16. How much physical assistance is given when it is:
    - maximal?
    - moderate?
    - slight?

17. How much verbal assistance is given when it is:
    - maximal?
    - moderate?
    - slight?

18. Why is it important to know how much time it takes the patient to eat?

Multidisciplinary Swallowing Program

Inservice Quiz

1. What is dysphagia?

   Dysphagia is a disorder characterized by difficulty with swallowing. Improper care of a patient with dysphagia may result in aspiration pneumonia or death.

2. List 3 signs/symptoms of potential swallowing problems.

   Signs/symptoms of swallowing problems (any 3):
   - facial weakness
        poor lip closure
        facial droop
        drooling
   - apraxia*
        difficulty chewing
        difficulty with simple lip and tongue movements
   - decreased sensation
        pocketing (food in cheek)
        biting cheek
        food falling out of mouth
   - decreased throat clearing ability and protective cough
   - choking
   - coughing before, during, or after swallowing
   - difficulty managing secretions (may need frequent suctioning)
   - difficulty swallowing thin liquids (such as water, coffee)
   - decreased mentation (confusion), which may result in inconsistent performance (may spit food out or hold food in mouth without swallowing)

3. List 3 "bad" foods for a patient with dysphagia.

   Bad foods:
   - thin liquids
        water
        coffee
        milk
   - spicy foods—may irritate throat
   - skins, seeds and nuts—may be easily aspirated
   - multiple consistencies (lumpy and watery, gelatin with fruit, minced meat, mixed vegetables)
   - foods that break up in the mouth
        cookies
        crackers
   - sticky, greasy, stringy or tough food

4. What is the *Toothette®* for?

   A *Toothette®* is used to stimulate the mouth *before* eating and to clean out the mouth at *the end of the meal.*

5. Into which side of the patient's mouth should you put food?

Put food into the strong side of the mouth (the side opposite from the weak arm and leg).

6. After putting food in the patient's mouth, how can you determine if the patient has swallowed?

After putting food in mouth, *look* for or *feel* for *swallow*. (See Appendix D, page 110, for instructions on how to feel for the swallow.)

7. What patient behaviors during feeding would tell you to stop feeding the patient?

Coughing or absence of swallowing should tell you to stop feeding the patient and to tell the registered nurse.

8. What are aspiration precautions?

Elevate head of bed 90 degrees. Support body as needed. Visually check mouth for pocketing and swallowing. Provide mouth care every 4 hours. Do not lower head of bed less than 45 degrees for at least 30 minutes after eating.

9. When and why should you use a "nosey cut-out cup?"

Nosey cut-out cups are used to *stop* patient from *tilting head up* and *back.* Use a nosey cup with patients who cough when drinking, *IF recommended by occupational therapist.*

10. When is it safe for a certified nursing assistant to feed a patient who has been receiving swallowing training from an occupational therapist and a speech-language pathologist?

Assistants should feed dysphagia patients ONLY when told to by occupational therapist or speech-language pathologist.

11. List 4 important facts given about the patient on the ATTENTION! sheet.

Four important facts about the patient found on the ATTENTION! sheet:
- dysphagia diet level
- position of patient
- patient needs for oral feeding
- adaptive equipment used

12. Who is responsible for filling out the Dysphagia Flow Sheet?

Only staff trained by the multidisciplinary swallowing team.

13. When should the Dysphagia Flow Sheet be completed?

Immediately following a meal.

14. What does the term *consistency not tolerated* refer to on the Dysphagia Flow Sheet?

Consistency not tolerated refers to the different food consistencies or types of liquids *not* tolerated by patient or which cause signs/symptoms of aspiration.

15. How are "Food%" and "cc" intake determined?

The trained staff person uses the method for calculating caloric intake and food percentages found in Appendixes H and I, pages 114-117. The amount of liquid volume consumed is determined by the normal values found on the Dysphagia Flow Sheet.

16. **How much physical assistance is given when it is:**

The amount of physical assistance given when it is:

- *Maximal* is 8 to 10 out of 10 attempts to complete the feeding/swallowing process, requiring the feeding aide to physically intervene in order for patient to be successful and safe.
- *Moderate* is 6 to 7 out of 10 attempts.
- *Slight* is 1 to 3 out of 10 attempts.

17. **How much verbal assistance is given when it is:**

The amount of verbal assistance given when it is:

- *Maximal* is 8 to 10 out of 10 attempts to complete the feeding/swallowing process, requiring the feeding aide to verbally intervene in order for patient to be successful and safe.
- *Moderate* is 6 to 7 out of 10 attempts.
- *Slight* is 1 to 3 out of 10 attempts.

18. **Why is it important to know how much time it takes the patient to eat?**

It is important to document the amount of eating time in order to work toward a functional time limit and to document improvement in physical endurance as it influences feeding.

3 ■ Assessment

Introduction

This chapter provides five filled-in sample forms, plus instructions for using the forms, to help the multidisciplinary swallowing team in recordkeeping, evaluation, and planning. Reproducible blank forms are located at the end of the chapter.

The forms include:

- Swallowing Screening (for use by nursing)
- Multidisciplinary Swallowing Team Treatment Plan
- Speech-Language Pathology Swallowing Evaluation
- Occupational Therapy Feeding Evaluation
- Dietary Nutritional Assessment

The chapter also includes guidelines:

- to help determine the level of severity of the patient's dysphagia
- to help determine whether the patient should be fed by oral or non-oral methods
- for conducting swallowing evaluations for patients who have a tracheostoma tube.

Completing the Swallowing Screening Form

This form is completed by a registered nurse as part of the initial nursing assessment of the patient. It is used to identify those patients who are suspected of having dysphagia, and to refer them to the appropriate multidisciplinary team members for further assessment.

Complete the form by checking off observed symptoms during the initial assessment, at mealtime, or when medicine is administered.

The screening is failed if *any* item is checked. The patient should be referred to speech-language pathology, occupational therapy, and dietary personnel.

Swallowing Screening

Patient's name ___S. C.___

___112656___   Room # ___20B___   Date ___10/5/xx___

Note to nursing staff

Complete this checklist as part of the initial nursing assessment for every patient. If the patient exhibits any one symptom, screening is failed.

- ☐ Difficult, labored swallowing
- ☒ Aspiration precautions
- ☒ Drooling
- ☐ Copious oral secretions
- ☐ Coughing, choking, strangling at meals
- ☐ Holding or pocketing of food in mouth
- ☐ Absence of chewing
- ☐ Food comes back at front of mouth
- ☒ Excessive throat clearing, gurgling voice
- ☐ Difficulty swallowing medications

☒ *Screening failed*   ☐ *Screening passed*

If screening is failed, please

- ☒ Notify speech pathology
- ☒ Notify occupational therapy
- ☒ Notify dietary

Nurse signature ___Sharon Jonas___

Date ___10-5-XX___

Completing the Multidisciplinary Swallowing Team Treatment Plan

This treatment plan is used to inform physicians and staff of team recommendations for patient care during the upcoming week. It should be filled out by the members of the team at the weekly team meeting and kept in the nursing section of the patient's chart. Below are some sample entries.

Nursing

Insure all medications are crushed and administered in applesauce.

Monitor weight weekly.

Dietary

Advance diet to Dysphagia Advanced.

Administer calorie count twice this week.

Speech-language pathology

Continue with oral-motor strengthening and bolus-control exercises.

Continue training patient, family, and staff in facilitative swallowing techniques.

Occupational therapy

Train patient in use of adaptive equipment.

Ensure proper patient positioning at mealtime.

Multidisciplinary Swallowing Team
Treatment Plan

Patient's name ____S. C._____

___112656___ Rm # _121_____ Age _75____ Date _10/7/xx_____

Dysphagia Dx ___mod.-sev.; oral pharyngeal dysphagia_____

Medical Dx ___R hemisphere CVA_____ Physician ___Dr. Jones_____

Current diet and method of intake ___gastrostomy tube feeding_____

Recommended diet/intake __Continue with same pending results of additional medical work·

Team members' signatures *Lori Marsden*   *J. Jones, M.D.*

Margaret Smith

Nursing

Administer tube feedings. Check for residuals. Elevate head of bed (HOB)
45 degrees. Mouth care every 4 hours.

Dietary

Monitor tube feedings. Adjust as needed with increased activity. Maintain
current weight as within ideal range.

Speech-language pathologist

Refer patient for videofluoroscopic swallowing study. Initiate oral-motor
exercises. Initiate laryngeal function exercises. Thermal stimulation.

Occupational therapist

To eat at least 25% of meals and consume 50% of all appropriate liquids
on each tray with 1:1 supervision within 30 minutes.

Completing the Speech-Language Pathology Swallowing Evaluation

This form is for clinical bedside administration. Whenever possible, additional assessment through videofluoroscopic, endoscopic, manometric or scintigraphic* studies is suggested. Voice and oral-motor evaluations are also recommended.

Review the dysphagia diagnosis, recommendations, and treatment plan at the multidisciplinary swallowing team meeting. Information obtained from this evaluation, along with assessments from other team members, is used to complete the "ATTENTION!" feeding/swallowing instruction sheet (see Chapter 7, pages 85, 89).

Many patients with mechanical dysphagia (as opposed to neurogenic dysphagia, the focus of this manual) have a tracheostoma tube (Groher 1984, p. 164). See page 41 for suggested procedures for evaluating patients with tracheostoma tubes.

Name and pertinent biographical information

Complete these items, using the patient's medical chart as a reference. The **diagnosis** refers to primary medical diagnosis associated with the patient's dysphagia. The **onset date** refers to the date of onset of the primary diagnosis (such as *CVA 12/1/89)* or the date that swallowing function was impaired.

Baseline

Discuss swallowing status existing prior to onset of current diagnosis (such as *swallowing reported to be within normal limits prior to this CVA*). This information can be obtained from medical records or verbal reports of patient, family, or staff.

History

Discuss pertinent hospitalization and medical history. Mention previous dysphagia treatment, if appropriate.

Presenting problem

Identify and specify the primary presenting problem or reason for referral (such as *food comes back out of mouth, coughs a lot at mealtime,* or *gets strangled on water*).

Current method of nutrition

Describe feeding method (such as tube or oral feeding) and diet consistency.

Objective

Use the checklists on pages 2 and 3 of the form to complete this portion of the evaluation.

If the patient's status is "NPO" (nothing by mouth) as determined by your chart review (and as stated on this form under Current Method of Nutrition), consult with the patient's physician prior to initiating trial or diagnostic oral intake.

If the patient is feeding orally, evaluate swallowing at mealtime, if possible, to get a realistic picture of the patient's functional swallowing ability.

Ask the patient to start with easily tolerated consistencies, such as thick liquids or pureed foods, and with small (½ teaspoon) amounts. Observe the patient with at least three boluses of each of the following consistencies: liquid, paste, and solid.

Oral preparatory and oral phase. Complete the checklist as you examine for difficulties in the oral stage of the swallow, involving lips, tongue, teeth, chewing, and oral cavity.

Velopharyngeal and pharyngeal phase. Continue the checklist as you identify symptoms involving the larynx, pharynx, soft palate, and cricopharyngeus. Note whether the patient can effectively cough and clear the throat. Esophageal peristalsis difficulties may also be noted here.

Clinical aspiration symptoms. Check those items associated with signs of possible aspiration and note whether they occurred before, during, or after swallow.

Assessment

Turn to page 3 of the form. Using the Dysphagia Functional Severity Levels guidelines (page 39), report the dysphagia **Diagnosis and Severity Level** in the space provided. Discuss the patient's **prognosis** for recovering partial or full swallowing function.

Circle the **consistencies tested.** Briefly indicate the patient's **ability to follow instructions,** overall level of **responsiveness,** and patient's **awareness of swallowing problem.**

Note whether a videofluoroscopic or scintigraphic study is indicated. A patient should be referred for one of these studies if:

- aspiration is present or suspected
- the patient's swallowing disorder has a pharyngeal origin or component (Logemann 1983)
- the facility policy requires this before proceeding with dysphagia rehabilitation.

A videofluoroscopic or scintigraphic study can also rule out silent aspiration.

Treatment plan

Indicate a plan of treatment which includes frequency (and duration, in some settings) of services. Describe the type of treatment needed. Suggestions can be found in Chapter 5.

Long-term goals

Specify the swallowing status the patient is expected to achieve by completion of treatment. Sample LTGs can be found in Chapter 5.

Short-term goals

Describe graduated, detailed skills leading to the LTGs that the patient is expected to develop as treatment progresses. See Chapter 5 for additional information and guidelines.

Speech-Language Pathology
Swallowing Evaluation

Patient's name __S. C.__

\# __112656__ Date __10/6/xx__ Age __75__ Sex __M__

Referring physician __Jones__ Admitted from __Home__

Dates of stay __n/a__

Diagnosis __Right hemisphere CVA__

Onset date __10/1/xx__

Other pertinent medical or surgical information __History of hypertension, aspiration__ __pneumonia 10/5/xx__

Baseline __swallowing within normal limits prior to CVA__

History __living independently at home with spouse; retired airline pilot__

Presenting problem ____

Current method of nutrition __gastrostomy tube placed 10/5/xx; receives tube feeding__

Objective: See evaluations, pages 2 and 3

Assessment: See evaluations, pages 2 and 3

Treatment plan __Obtain videofluoroscopic swallowing study. Initiate speech-language__ __pathology treatment daily.__

Long term goal(s) __Determine potential for safe adequate oral intake and introduce__ __food liquid by mouth, if indicated.__

Short term goal(s) __Further medical evaluation by videofluoroscopic swallowing study.__ __Improved labial and lingual strength and range of motion; improved laryngeal__ __functioning; increased speed and consistency of swallow reflex with thermal__ __stimulation.__

Speech-language pathologist _Lori Marsden_

Physician's name __J. Jones, M.D.__

Signature _J. Jones, M.D._

Date __10/6/xx__ Telephone __999-4561__

Speech-language Pathology
Swallowing Evaluation (page 2)

Patient's name ___S. C._____ Date ___10/6/xx_____

Oral Preparatory and Oral Phase

Symptoms exhibited	*Impairment*
☒ food, liquid leaks from mouth	☒ reduced labial closure
☒ separation of food in mouth, loss of bolus . . . . control, may aspirate before swallow (periodicaly)	☒ reduced lingual control
☒ food falls into lateral sulcus ..left.	☒ reduced buccal tension
☐ food remains on tongue or hard palate	☐ incomplete tongue-to-palate contact
☒ residue not felt by patient, ... may aspirate before swallow	☒ reduced oral sensitivity
☐ food remains on tongue, teeth; . . . . bolus does not go back in mouth	☐ reduced anterior to posterior lingual movement
☐ slow oral transit	☐ reduced mastication and lingual movement, delayed reflex
☐ reduced chewing, delayed or absent . . . . rotary chewing	☐ poor dental status; reduced mandibular control, strength

Velopharyngeal and Pharyngeal Phase

Symptoms exhibited	*Impairment*
☐ poor or absent elevation of hyoid, ... thyroid cartilage	☐ absent reflex, possible loss of airway protection, hesitation in valleculae
☐ delayed elevation of hyoid, thyroid	☐ hesitation in valleculae
☒ repeated swallows per bolus	☒ reduced pharyngeal peristalsis
☐ complains of discomfort high in throat	☐ unilateral pharyngeal paralysis; residue of material on 1 side of valleculae
☐ complains of discomfort low in throat	☐ cricopharyngeal dysfunction or reduced esophageal peristalsis
☒ gurgly voice quality	☒ decreased laryngeal elevation
☐ gag reflex	(present) (absent)
☒ volitional cough	(productive) (nonproductive)
☒ clear throat	(productive) (nonproductive)
☐ expectoration of material after swallow	☐ reduced pharyngeal peristalsis; residue of material in valleculae; residue of material in pyriform sinus

Speech-language Pathology
Swallowing Evaluation (page 3)

Clinical Aspiration Symptoms

Symptoms exhibited	*Impairment*
☒ coughing, choking *before* swallow	☒ delayed or absent reflex; reduced lingual coordination to form bolus
☐ coughing, choking *during* swallow	☐ reduced vocal cord closure
☒ coughing, choking *after* swallow, ... gurgly voice after swallow	☒ decreased laryngeal elevation, cricopharyngeal dysfunction, collection of material in pyriform sinuses
☐ food doesn't go down, food coughed up	☐ absent swallow reflex
☐ excessive, copious secretions	☐ aspiration
☐ nasal or oral regurgitation; coughing, ... choking after swallow; complains of fullness around area of sternum	☐ esophageal or pharyngeal obstruction, fistula, diverticulum, velopharyngeal obstruction

Diagnosis and Severity Level

Moderate-to-severe oral pharyngeal dysphagia, complicated by attention and

mental status.

Prognosis Pending results of videofluoroscopic swallow study; patient to remain

in NPO currently.

Consistencies tested—(liquid, paste,) solid

Ability to follow instructions_____Fair

Responsiveness_____Fair to good

Awareness of problem_____Fair

Videofluoroscopic study indicated _____Yes

Completing the Occupational Therapy
Feeding Evaluation

Each item on the evaluation form is listed below, accompanied by instructions for completion. Information obtained from this evaluation is used to complete the "ATTENTION!" feeding/swallowing instruction sheet (see Chapter 7, pages 85, 89).

Name and pertinent biographical information

Complete these items using the patient's medical chart as a reference. **Diagnosis** refers to the primary medical diagnosis associated with the patient's feeding problem, as well as diagnoses that may influence outcome of evaluation and treatment. **Onset date** refers to the date of the diagnosis directly associated with the feeding problem (such as *CVA, 12/1/89*).

Baseline

Use information obtained from medical records or verbal reports from physician, patient, family, or staff to determine pre-injury baseline feeding status.

Presenting problem

Identify and specify the primary presenting problem (such as *patient consistently spills, drops food on lap*) secondary to sensory loss and neglect.

Findings pertinent to feeding

This section reviews how the following factors influence feeding success.

Physical limitations. Identify upper- and lower-body limitations affecting body positioning, and discuss effective use of upper extremities. Indicate the type of hand-to-mouth and grasp/release patterns used by the patient.

Perceptual deficits. Refers to the patient's spatial awareness, unilateral neglect, sensory-motor planning deficits, and tactile deficits.

Cognition. Identify cognitive limitations such as functional communication, orientation, memory, attention span, ability to follow instructions, and judgment or reasoning abilities.

Vision and hearing. Identify the patient's visual tracking ability and visual field deficits; estimate the patient's functional hearing ability.

Motivation. Discuss the patient's interest and cooperation in feeding.

Amount of physical assistance required. Specify amount and kind of physical assistance required in order for the patient to safely complete a meal.

Amount of verbal assistance required. Specify amount and type of verbal assistance or cuing necessary for the patient to safely complete a meal.

Amount of time required. Describe the amount of time expressed in minutes taken to consume an adequate portion (75 percent) of the meal.

Swallowing difficulties. Describe the patient's tolerance of food consistencies in the swallowing process (such as *swallowed with difficulty, some coughing after swallowing,* or *choking, strangling with all consistencies*).

Recommendations and plans

The contents of this section should be discussed at the multidisciplinary swallowing team meeting.

Realistic goals. Specify short- and long-term functional goals. (Refer to Chapter 5 for assistance with goal specifications.)

Adaptive equipment necessary. List the type of feeding utensils, equipment, and positioning devices needed to facilitate more efficient feeding.

Setup or special assistance. Specify body positioning, placement of the patient in relation to the person assisting with feeding, and type of physical and verbal assistance to be given during the meal.

Approach

Indicate specific instructions to be given to the patient during the feeding and swallowing process (such as *remember to place the spoonful of food on the stronger* [or *left*] *side of your mouth*). Also discuss the amount and type of verbal praise or reinforcement the patient needs to promote greater independence.

Date to begin program

Specify the date the patient begins a particular feeding program (such as a restorative feeding class or individual occupational therapy feeding).

Occupational Therapy Feeding Evaluation

Patient's name ___S. C.___

\# ___112656___ Date ___11/3/xx___ Age ___75___ Sex ___M___

Referring physician ___Dr. Jones___ Admitted from ___General Hospital___

Dates of stay ___10/1/xx – 11/2/xx___

Diagnosis ___(R) CVA with (L) side involvement___

Onset date ___10/1/xx___

Other pertinent medical or surgical information ___Recurring C-difficile Colitis, CHF, Aspiration___
___pneumonia, gastrostomy tube placement 10/5/xx; videofluoroscopic study 10/7/xx;___
___Received ST for swallowing therapy, PT and OT.___

Baseline ___Able to manage all food consistency and eat independently prior to CVA.___
___NPO except for trial oral feeding by ST and OT.___

Presenting problem ___Dysphagia with perceptual deficits, unable to eat safely and___
___independently.___

Findings pertinent to feeding

Physical limitations ___Wheelchair bound with mild spastic left upper extremity and mild___
___spasticity in left lower extremity.___

Perceptual deficits ___Severe left side neglect with moderate perceptual deficits, depth___
___perception, body image, and tactile-kinesthetic awareness, motor apraxia.___

Cognition ___Alert. Not consistently oriented to place, time or situation. Moderately___
___impaired short-term memory. Exhibits short attention span, poor judgment/reason-___
___ing abilities and inconsistently follows direction.___

Vision and hearing ___Poor vision. Left hemianopia with poor visual-motor skills___
___(tracking/scanning) to left visual field. Hearing within functional limits.___
___Needs directions repeated due to poor attention span.___

Motivation ___Good for eating.___

Amount of physical assistance required ___Minimal physical assistance required once tray___
___is set up.___

Occupational Therapy Feeding Evaluation
(page 2)

Amount of verbal assistance required Moderate cuing needed to alternate sip – bite – sip; take 1/2 to 1 teaspoon of food; cough; clear voice and relax.

Amount of time required ± 45 minutes for 25% to 50% of food and 9 to 13 ounces of juice and milk. He tires after 15 to 20 minutes with swallowing showing delay up to 7 seconds.

Swallowing difficulties Delayed swallow with increased delay occurring with being tired. Uses body movements to assist swallowing when tired.

Recommendations and plans

Realistic goals To eat at least 50% of each meal and consume all appropriate liquids on each tray with 1:1 supervision within 30 minutes.

Adaptive equipment necessary Straw holder

Setup or special assistance Place straw in straw holder position food in body midline and drink to the right of plate. Have tissue to right on table with wastebasket to his right. Interrupt extraneous movement verbally and physically if necessary.

Approach Verbally cue him to sip – take 1/2 to 1 tsp. bite – sip. Must swallow after each bolus and count the seconds. Have him say "all clear" or talk after sequence and to clear if needed. Should not take deep breaths with any food or liquid in mouth.

Date to begin program 11/3/xx

Therapist's signature *Marci Lawson*

Date 11- 3 -xx

Attending physician's signature J. Jones, M.D.

Date 11/3/xx

Completing the Dietary Nutritional Assessment

A nutritional assessment is administered for every patient to determine the patient's current nutritional status, to identify any nutritional problems, and to develop a plan of action.

Basic chart information

This includes admission date, birth date, patient's name, physician, patient number, and room number. Also listed here are the **diet order** (including any nutritional supplements ordered) and **current** and **relevant past diagnoses** (consider relevancy of diet order to diagnoses).

Patient's current physical and mental status

Use this checklist to indicate presence or absence of impairments in the listed areas.

Pertinent medications

Include vitamin and mineral supplements.

Laboratory results

List those results which have nutritional significance.

Diet history

Identify aspects of the patient's history which have nutritional implications. This can include patient's past weight history from the patient and/or family, or other significant information obtained from the patient's medical history, such as food allergies or preferences.

Normal food and fluid patterns/Food allergies

Include what, if any, special diets the patient had been on previously.

Observation of dietary intake in facility

This data may be recorded in percentage or caloric form. Also, document any major food group(s) not consumed.

Estimated nutritional needs

Determine and record weight in pounds and kilograms. Determine and record height in inches and centimeters. Determine desirable weight range.

Estimated caloric needs

Basal energy expenditures (BEE.) Circle **male** or **female,** and use the formula for that gender to calculate the basal energy expenditure. To do this, enter the calculations for weight in kilograms and height in centimeters on the appropriate lines. Enter patient's age.

Now complete the math functions. Multiply the designated number by the patient's weight in kilograms, and enter this figure in the bracket above. Do the same with the calculations using height in centimeters and age. After all calculations have been entered in brackets, complete the addition and subtraction to determine the calories needed for basal energy expenditure.

Total caloric needs. Circle an activity factor based on the patient's activity pattern. If the patient has an infection or injury, circle an injury factor and record the specific infection or injury in the margin. If the patient does not have an injury or infection, write 0 (or *none*). Enter these factors and the BEE calculation and complete the math functions. This calculation represents the patient's total daily energy expenditure (TDE).

Energy for weight gain or loss. Calculate the patient's percentage above or below desirable body weight. Use the calories needed for TDE and add or subtract 500 calories per day for weight gain or loss. List this figure as **total caloric needs.**

Estimated protein needs

Choose a protein requirement factor and multiply it by the body weight in kilograms. This gives the grams of protein needed. The protein requirement factor is often the same as the injury factor used in estimating caloric needs.

Estimated fluid needs

Multiply the current weight in kilograms by 30 cc. This gives the fluid requirement. (For those patients with a diagnosis of **congestive heart failure,** multiply by 25 cc/ kilogram. For those patients who have a **urinary tract infection** or recurrent urinary tract infections, multiply by 40 cc/kilogram.)

An additional 500-1500 cc may be needed if diarrhea, vomiting, or fever is noted.

Evaluation/Conclusions

When specific nutritional problems (needs) are identified, the nutritional care plan will include a plan of action (intervention) with an expected outcome (goal). When no nutritional problems are identified, an ongoing plan to provide and monitor adequate nutrition will be provided.

Preliminary nutritional care plan

Review the assessment at least quarterly, and more often when indicated by a change in patient status. Write a progress note after each review. This note will comment on progress of identified problems, identify new problems as they arise, or comment on current status. The care plan should be updated with each change in patient status.

Dietary Nutritional Assessment

Patient

Name __Johnson, Diane__ Patient no. __6320__

Room no._____ Adm. date __1/15/xx__ Sex __F__ Birth date __7/3/xx__ Age __59__

Physician __Kildare__

Diet order __Pureed diet as tolerated. Ensure 8 oz TID__

Current diagnoses __Rt hemisphere CVA__

Relevant past diagnoses __Hx of hypertension; Hypothyroidism__

Patient Status

Impaired	Yes	No
Ability to feed self	☐	☐
Chewing	☐	☐
Swallowing	☐	☐
Taste	☐	☐
Mobility	☐	☐
Vision	☐	☐
Hearing	☐	☐
Communicating skills	☐	☐
Bowel	☐	☐
Bladder	☐	☐
Mental abilities	☐	☐
Appetite	☐	☐
Presence of edema	☐	☐
Presence of decubitus	☐	☐

Decubitus stage/location _____

Pertinent medications

Order date __1/15/xx--Synthroid__

Applicable laboratory data

Date __1/7/xx__ (in hospital)

Test results __hgb 12.3 hct 38.2__
__albumin 3.7__
__electrolytes WNL__

Diet history

Normal food and fluid patterns __Prior to stroke ate foods from all major food groups. No food dislikes or intolerances. Since CVA has been able to tolerate small volume pureed foods, essentially no liquids.__

Food allergies __No known food allergies.__

Dietary Nutritional Assessment (page 2)

Observation of dietary intake in facility

Meals observed __Breakfast 1/16/xx; Dinner 1/17/xx__

Dining location __Room__

Ability to chew/swallow solid foods __Chewing ability very limited, much difficulty in__ __swallowing. Pt very tired and discouraged over inability to eat.__

Ability to consume thick and thin liquids __Pt strangled when trying to drink orange juice.__ __Tried Ensure since it is thicker. Pt. still choked and became frightened.__

Type and amount of assistance needed __Currently pt needs total assistance with feeding__ __even though she is able to handle spoon herself she does not try to feed herself.__

Percentage intake of meal observed: ____25__ % Food ____10__ % Fluids

Supplemental feedings: (List enteral feedings given, summary of what the feedings provide)
__Ensure 8 oz TID provides 760 calories, 27 grams of protein. However, pt__ __consuming less than 10% at this time.__

Name __M. S.__

Physician __Kildare__

Record # __6320__   Rm # __201-B__

Estimated nutritional needs

Weight __163__ lbs __74__ kg. (Weight in kg. = weight in lbs. x 2.2)   Desirable weight: _____ Low

Height __65__ inches __165__ cm. (Height in cm. = height in inches x 2.54)   Desirable weight: _____ High

Estimated caloric needs

Female: B.E.E. = 655 + __710__ + __297__ − __277__ = __1385__
                (9.6 x kg)   (1.7 x cm)   (4.7 x age)   Kcal

Male: B.E.E. = 66 + _____ + _____ − _____ = _____
                (13.7 x kg)   (5 x cm)   (6.8 x age)   Kcal

Total caloric needs: __1385__ x __1.3__ x __---__ = __1800__
                B.E.E.   Activity   Injury/decub   Kcal

Pt is allowed 30% above
IBW, she has reserves
to draw on, could manage on reduced calorie level.   __-500__
Add or subtract 500 Kcal for 1# gain or loss per week.   __1300__ calories, minimum

Activity		Injury		Infection		Decub	
Confined to bed	= 1.2	Minor surgery	= 1.1	Mild	= 1.2	Stage II	= 1.2
Out of bed	= 1.3	Major surgery	= 1.2	Mod	= 1.4	Stage III	= 1.4
Active	= 1.5	Skeletal trauma	= 1.35	Severe	= 1.6	Stage IV	= 1.6
Comatose for years	= 1.1						

Dietary Nutritional Assessment (page 3)

Estimated protein needs

<u> 74 </u> x <u> .8 - 1.0 </u> = <u> 60-74 </u>   Normal: .8 to 1.0/kg

wt/kg   Pro. factor   grams pro   Decub: 1.2 to 1.5/kg

Estimated Fluid Needs

<u> 74 </u> x 30 cc = <u> 2590 </u>   25 cc/kg for CHF

wt/kg   cc's fluid   40 cc/kg for UTI

Evaluation/conclusions

Pt appears well nourished; lab data WNL. Wt is 30% above IBW with no other nutritional risk factors, so could manage on 1300 calories per day until she reached top of IBW range (112-138#) as long as she does not lose too fast. Major concern is reaching that level of calories and maintaining hydration when she is unable to consume liquids orally. Recommend changing supplement to Ensure Plus 4 oz TID, thickened to consistency patient can tolerate.

Preliminary nutritional care plan

Date	Problem	Outcome/goal	Plan
1/18/xx	Patient consuming only 20% of pureed diet.	Pt will consume 50% of Dysphagia Pureed Diet within 1 week.	Pt will be fed by trained therapist
	Pt fluid intake in-adequate to maintain hydration (needs 2000 cc per day)	Pt will consume 75% of thickened supplement within one week.	I + 0 Recommend physician consider IV support Recommend Ensure Plus 4 oz TID, thickened to consistency pt can tolerate.

Laura James
Signature of dietitian/dietary manager

Date <u> 1/18/xx </u>

Name <u> M.S. </u>

Physician <u> Kildare </u>

Record # <u> 6320 </u>   Rm # <u> 201-B </u>

Dysphagia Functional Severity Levels

The following guidelines are provided to facilitate determination of severity of dysphagia based on the patient's current level of functioning during the feeding-swallowing process.

Severe, nonfunctional

- Patient receives nothing by mouth (NPO).
- All nourishment taken by non-oral (enteral) feedings.
- In some cases, trial diagnostic oral intake, in small amounts, is given by speech-language pathologist or occupational therapist, with physician's orders.

Moderately severe, functionally impaired

- Patient has inconsistent or insufficient oral intake.
- Nonoral feedings may be altered or held for trial periods.
- Team decides at end of week whether to continue oral intake or return to nonoral feedings.
- Patient needs assistance and supervision at all times by nursing staff and dysphagia team.

Moderate, functionally impaired

- Patient's oral intake is becoming more consistent with prescribed dysphagia diet and use of facilitative techniques.
- Nonoral feedings may be altered or held for trial one- to two-week periods.
- Dysphagia team working on additional deletion or modification of diet items and facilitating techniques.
- Patient continues to receive one-on-one assistance or supervision.
- Nursing staff are feeders, following recommendations of dysphagia team.

Mild-moderate, approaching functional level

- Patient's oral intake is fairly consistent with prescribed dysphagia diet and use of facilitation techniques.
- Non-oral feedings may be held or discontinued.
- Patient may continue to have difficulty with certain consistencies, such as thin liquids.
- Patient continues to need some assistance by nursing, and receives supervision at each meal.
- Self-feeding instruction is started by occupational therapy if patient has sufficient upper extremity function.

Mild, functional but reduced

- Patient receives pureed, mechanical soft, or regular diet, with some restrictions. Items such as thin liquids, or solids that tend to crumble or break apart, may be omitted if patient has difficulty with them.
- Patient may still need to use facilitating techniques to swallow safely.
- Patient may continue to require occasional supervision, reminders, or assistance with compensatory techniques.
- Patient may be advanced to restorative feeding program or supervised feeding group.

Minimal, functional but reduced

- Patient consumes mechanical soft or regular diet with few or no restricted items.
- Patient is independent and needs no supervision.
- Patient may continue to have periodic difficulty with certain items such as thin liquids.

Normal, functional, and adequate

- Patient independently consumes all food and liquid consistencies safely and efficiently.
- Swallowing is within normal limits.

(These levels and descriptions have been developed based on guidelines published in *Clinical Evaluation of Dysphagia,* Rehabilitation Institute of Chicago, 1986, and J. S. Steefel's *Dysphagia Rehabilitation for Neurologically Impaired Adults,* Charles C. Thomas, 1981.)

Guidelines for Determining Oral vs. Non-Oral Feeding

Aspiration

Any patient who is aspirating significantly (more than 10 percent of each bolus, regardless of consistency) should not be feeding orally. The patient who is aware of the aspiration and aspirates more than 10 percent of each bolus will eliminate that consistency from the diet by no longer attempting to eat it (Logemann et al. 1980).

The patient who is unaware of the aspiration will continue to eat and drink despite aspiration of significant amounts. This percentage is best determined by videofluoroscopic swallowing studies (Logemann et al. 1980).

Time

Any patient who is taking more than 10 seconds to eat every bolus of food or liquid (of each consistency) is unlikely to be able to maintain adequate nutrition with oral intake alone. If the patient's function is borderline (patient takes approximately 10 seconds to eat each bolus), the dietitian may provide diet supplements to increase the caloric content of foods eaten orally. These patients would be diagnosed as having moderately severe to severe dysphagia (Logemann, et al. 1980).

Adequacy of intake

Any patient who is unable to take sufficient oral feedings to maintain adequate nutritional status will need non-oral feedings. The sufficiency of oral intake is determined by comparing the patient's estimated needs for calories, protein, and fluid to the calculation of actual intake.

The patient's estimated needs for calories, protein, and fluid are listed on the initial nutritional assessment.

Percentage intake of all meals and supplements will be recorded by the person assisting or monitoring the feeding. Percentage intake charts are provided for each level of the diet.

The patient's ability to consume adequate fluids without symptoms of aspiration (choking, coughing or strangling) will also be considered.

Enteral feeding*/supplementation recommendations may be made if one or more of the following situations occurs:

- Intake of food and fluid provided on any level of the diet is below 50 percent for three consecutive days. At this point the strategy may be to resume enteral feedings in the evening and at night, and allow the patient to continue rehabilitative efforts during the day.

- Total calories consumed are inadequate to meet estimated caloric needs after two consecutive calorie counts, or a significant increase in intake has not occurred in the past week.

- Patient has experienced significant weight loss prior to being placed on the dysphagia protocol. Consider the weight loss to be significant if the patient has lost more than 5 percent of total body weight during the previous month, or more than 7½ percent of total body weight in the previous three months.

Evaluating Patients Who Have a Tracheostoma Tube

For those individuals with tracheostoma tubes, the following methods of evaluation are recommended (Logemann 1983; Groher 1984; Langley 1987). A related method described by Cameron et al. (1973) has also been included.

It should be noted that the introduction of oral intake in individuals with cuffed tracheostoma tubes is somewhat controversial. A number of authors suggest that oral intake be postponed or restricted when an individual's respiratory status necessitates an inflated cuff (Bonanno 1971; Fleming 1984; Groher 1984). Because of this, *the patient's physician should be consulted on the advisability of deflating the patient's tracheostoma tube cuff prior to administering a swallowing evaluation.* Tracheostoma tubes can restrict the elevation and tilting of the larynx during the swallow and an inflated cuff may irritate the trachea during laryngeal elevation (Logemann 1983; Groher 1984; Nash 1988).

If a decision is made to deflate the cuff, it is important to suction the patient well in the oral cavity and in the trachea above the cuff. This suctioning should be performed by trained nursing, respiratory, or physical therapy staff.

Next, deflate the cuff and again suction the patient well. Plug the tube for several seconds to insure the patient's ability to breathe through the larynx. When the tube is occluded with a finger, air should pass around the tube and through the larynx (Logemann 1983, p. 102). If the diameter of the tracheostoma tube is such that it occludes much of the tracheal lumen, occlusion of the tracheostoma tube will not allow a sufficient amount of pulmonary air to reach the larynx. This blockage can be alleviated by employing a smaller diameter or fenestrated tube (Groher 1984, p. 166) to allow for greater air flow (Logemann 1983, p. 104).

To establish tracheal pressure, plug or occlude the tracheostoma tube during each swallow. Practice dry swallows first. Ice chips can then be attempted. To check for aspiration, use a stimulus that is dyed with a contrasting color that can be detected in the trachea (such as methylene blue, 0.5 ml in 30 ml water) (Groher 1984, p. 97). The trachea should be suctioned periodically for evidence of the blue coloring solution, which is an indicator of aspiration (Cameron et al. 1973; Groher 1984).

In a similar procedure, Cameron used an Evans blue dye test to assess for aspiration in 61 patients with tracheostomies. Here, four drops of the blue dye are placed on the patient's tongue every four hours. When routine tracheostomy care is performed, evidence of dye in the trachea is considered to be indicative of aspiration. In this study, 69 percent of the patients demonstrated evidence of aspiration with an average time of seven hours to test positive. However, there were no significant differences related to the presence of a nasogastric tube or degree of patient responsiveness, or among patients using cuffed versus uncuffed tracheostoma tubes.

Swallowing Screening

Patient's name _____

_____ Room # _____ Date _____

Note to nursing staff

Complete this checklist as part of the initial nursing assessment for every patient. If the patient exhibits any one symptom, screening is failed.

- ☐ Difficult, labored swallowing
- ☐ Aspiration precautions
- ☐ Drooling
- ☐ Copious oral secretions
- ☐ Coughing, choking, strangling at meals
- ☐ Holding or pocketing of food in mouth
- ☐ Absence of chewing
- ☐ Food comes back at front of mouth
- ☐ Excessive throat clearing, gurgling voice
- ☐ Difficulty swallowing medications

☐ *Screening failed*   ☐ *Screening passed*

If screening is failed, please

- ☐ Notify speech pathology
- ☐ Notify occupational therapy
- ☐ Notify dietary

Nurse signature_____

Date _____

Multidisciplinary Swallowing Team
Treatment Plan

Patient's name _____

\# _____ Rm # _____ Age _____ Date _____

Dysphagia Dx _____

Medical Dx _____ Physician _____

Current diet and method of intake _____

Recommended diet/intake _____

Team members' signatures _____

_____

Nursing

Dietary

Speech-language pathologist

Occupational therapist

Speech-Language Pathology
Swallowing Evaluation

Patient's name _____

_____ Date _____ Age _____ Sex _____

Referring physician _____ Admitted from _____

Dates of stay _____

Diagnosis _____

Onset date _____

Other pertinent medical or surgical information_____

_____

_____

Baseline _____

History_____

_____

Presenting problem _____

_____

Current method of nutrition _____

_____

Objective: See evaluations, pages 2 and 3

Assessment: See evaluations, pages 2 and 3

Treatment plan _____

_____

_____

Long term goal(s)_____

_____

_____

Short term goal(s) _____

_____

_____

_____

_____

Speech-language pathologist _____

Physician's name _____

Signature _____

Date _____Telephone _____

Speech-language Pathology
Swallowing Evaluation (page 2)

Patient's name _____ Date _____

Oral Preparatory and Oral Phase

Symptoms exhibited	Impairment
☐ food, liquid leaks from mouth	☐ reduced labial closure
☐ separation of food in mouth, loss of bolus . . . . control, may aspirate before swallow	☐ reduced lingual control
☐ food falls into lateral sulcus . . . . , ...	☐ reduced buccal tension
☐ food remains on tongue or hard palate	☐ incomplete tongue-to-palate contact
☐ residue not felt by patient, ... may aspirate before swallow	☐ reduced oral sensitivity
☐ food remains on tongue, teeth; . . . . bolus does not go back in mouth	☐ reduced anterior to posterior lingual movement
☐ slow oral transit	☐ reduced mastication and lingual movement, delayed reflex
☐ reduced chewing, delayed or absent . . . . rotary chewing	☐ poor dental status; reduced mandibular control, strength

Velopharyngeal and Pharyngeal Phase

Symptoms exhibited	Impairment
☐ poor or absent elevation of hyoid, ... thyroid cartilage	☐ absent reflex, possible loss of airway protection, hesitation in valleculae
☐ delayed elevation of hyoid, thyroid	☐ hesitation in valleculae
☐ repeated swallows per bolus	☐ reduced pharyngeal peristalsis
☐ complains of discomfort high in throat	☐ unilateral pharyngeal paralysis; residue of material on 1 side of valleculae
☐ complains of discomfort low in throat	☐ cricopharyngeal dysfunction or reduced esophageal peristalsis
☐ gurgly voice quality	☐ decreased laryngeal elevation
☐ gag reflex	(present) (absent)
☐ volitional cough	(productive) (nonproductive)
☐ clear throat	(productive) (nonproductive)
☐ expectoration of material after swallow	☐ reduced pharyngeal peristalsis; residue of material in valleculae; residue of material in pyriform sinus

Speech-language Pathology
Swallowing Evaluation (page 3)

Clinical Aspiration Symptoms

Symptoms exhibited	*Impairment*
☐ coughing, choking *before* swallow	☐ delayed or absent reflex; reduced lingual coordination to form bolus
☐ coughing, choking *during* swallow	☐ reduced vocal cord closure
☐ coughing, choking *after* swallow, ... gurgly voice after swallow	☐ decreased laryngeal elevation, cricopharyngeal dysfunction, collection of material in pyriform sinuses
☐ food doesn't go down, food coughed up	☐ absent swallow reflex
☐ excessive, copious secretions	☐ aspiration
☐ nasal or oral regurgitation; coughing, ... choking after swallow; complains of fullness around area of sternum	☐ esophageal or pharyngeal obstruction, fistula, diverticulum, velopharyngeal obstruction

Diagnosis and Severity Level

_____

_____

_____

Prognosis _____

_____

Consistencies tested—liquid, paste, solid

Ability to follow instructions_____

_____

Responsiveness_____

_____

Awareness of problem_____

_____

Videofluoroscopic study indicated _____

_____

Occupational Therapy Feeding Evaluation

Patient's name _____

\# _____ Date _____ Age _____ Sex_____

Referring physician _____ Admitted from_____

Dates of stay _____

Diagnosis_____

Onset date _____

Other pertinent medical or surgical information _____

_____

_____

_____

Baseline_____

_____

Presenting problem_____

_____

Findings pertinent to feeding

Physical limitations_____

_____

_____

Perceptual deficits _____

_____

_____

Cognition _____

_____

_____

_____

Vision and hearing _____

_____

_____

_____

Motivation _____

_____

_____

Amount of physical assistance required _____

_____

Occupational Therapy Feeding Evaluation

(page 2)

Amount of verbal assistance required _____

_____

_____

Amount of time required _____

_____

_____

Swallowing difficulties _____

_____

_____

Recommendations and plans

Realistic goals _____

_____

_____

_____

Adaptive equipment necessary _____

_____

_____

_____

Setup or special assistance _____

_____

_____

_____

Approach _____

_____

_____

_____

_____

Date to begin program _____

Therapist's signature _____

Date _____

Attending physician's signature _____

Date _____

Dietary Nutritional Assessment

Patient

Name _____ Patient no. _____

Room no. _____ Adm. date _____ Sex _____ Birth date _____ Age _____

Physician _____

Diet order _____

_____

Current diagnoses _____

_____

Relevant past diagnoses _____

_____

Patient Status

Impaired	Yes	No
Ability to feed self	☐	☐
Chewing	☐	☐
Swallowing	☐	☐
Taste	☐	☐
Mobility	☐	☐
Vision	☐	☐
Hearing	☐	☐
Communicating skills	☐	☐
Bowel	☐	☐
Bladder	☐	☐
Mental abilities	☐	☐
Appetite	☐	☐
Presence of edema	☐	☐
Presence of decubitus	☐	☐

Decubitus stage/location _____

_____

Pertinent medications

Order date _____

_____

_____

_____

_____

_____

_____

Applicable laboratory data

Date _____

Test results _____

_____

_____

_____

_____

_____

Diet history

Normal food and fluid patterns _____

_____

_____

Food allergies _____

Dietary Nutritional Assessment (page 2)

Observation of dietary intake in facility

Meals observed _____

Dining location _____

Ability to chew/swallow solid foods_____

_____

Ability to consume thick and thin liquids _____

_____

Type and amount of assistance needed _____

_____

Percentage intake of meal observed: _____% Food _____% Fluids

Supplemental feedings: (List enteral feedings given, summary of what the feedings provide)

_____

_____

_____

Name _____

Physician _____

Record # _____ Rm # _____

Estimated nutritional needs

Weight _____ lbs _____ kg. (Weight in kg. = weight in lbs. x 2.2) Desirable weight: _____ Low

Height _____ inches _____ cm. (Height in cm. = height in inches x 2.54) Desirable weight: _____ High

Estimated caloric needs

Female: B.E.E. = 655 + _____ + _____ − _____ = _____
                        (9.6 x kg)   (1.7 x cm)   (4.7 x age)   Kcal

Male: B.E.E. = 66 + _____ + _____ − _____ = _____
                        (13.7 x kg)   (5 x cm)   (6.8 x age)   Kcal

Total caloric needs: _____ x _____ x _____ = _____
                           B.E.E.   Activity   Injury/decub   Kcal

Add or subtract 500 Kcal for 1# gain or loss per week.

Activity		Injury		Infection		Decub	
Confined to bed	= 1.2	Minor surgery	= 1.1	Mild	= 1.2	Stage II	= 1.2
Out of bed	= 1.3	Major surgery	= 1.2	Mod	= 1.4	Stage III	= 1.4
Active	= 1.5	Skeletal trauma	= 1.35	Severe	= 1.6	Stage IV	= 1.6
Comatose for years	= 1.1						

Dietary Nutritional Assessment (page 3)

Estimated protein needs

_____ x _____ = _____   Normal: .8 to 1.0/kg

wt/kg   Pro. factor   grams pro   Decub: 1.2 to 1.5/kg

Estimated Fluid Needs

_____ x 30 cc = _____   25 cc/kg for CHF

wt/kg   cc's fluid   40 cc/kg for UTI

Evaluation/conclusions

_____
_____
_____
_____
_____
_____
_____
_____
_____

Preliminary nutritional care plan

Date	Problem	Outcome/goal	Plan

Signature of dietitian/dietary manager

Date _____

Name _____

Physician _____ _____

Record # _____ Rm # _____

4 ■ Dysphagia Diets, Consistencies, and Recipes

Dysphagia Diets

The following diets are designed as beginning or intermediate steps in a short-term, progressive rehabilitation program for patients with dysphagia. They provide the appropriate consistency of foods and liquids that allow the patient to swallow safely.

At first, some patients who receive these diets are able to consume only small quantities of food and *very* small volumes of fluid. Thus, weight loss and dehydration can occur rapidly. Many patients will need to receive enteral feedings until able to consume enough orally to maintain hydration and prevent significant weight loss.

The Level 2 dysphagia diet provides 75 percent to 100 percent of recommended caloric levels, 130 percent to 150 percent of recommended levels of protein, and 65 percent or more of the U.S. Recommended Daily Allowance of vitamins and minerals. How well the diet meets the needs of the individual patient depends upon the patient's gender and size and—*most importantly*—the actual intake of the diet.

Levels 3, 4, and 5 are adequate in all nutrients except water. Fluid will not be adequate until patient is able to consume at least one quart of actual fluids per day.

Classification of Liquids for Dysphagia Diets

Liquids in dysphagia diets are classified according to how much body or "thickness" they have. Generally, thick liquids are easier to control—presenting a lesser risk of aspiration—than are thin liquids. This chart lists examples of liquids classified as **thin** and **medium.** For examples of **thick** liquids, see *Level 1 Dysphagia Diet* on page 56.

Thin Liquids

	Recommended	Not allowed
Milk products	Milk (if so specified)	Milk (if not allowed)
Soups	Broth	
Beverages	Coffee, tea, fruit juices (such as apple juice, orange juice, grapefruit juice)	Soda
Miscellaneous	Gelatin, water	

Note: Milk tends to increase phlegm production in some individuals. For that reason, do not automatically include milk with thin liquids. Also, consider using cold thin liquids as they provide added sensory stimulation.

Medium Liquids

	Recommended	Not allowed
Milk products	Eggnog, milkshake	Milk which has not been thickened
Fruit juices	Nectar, juice frappe, tomato juice	Puree fruit, thin juices (such as apple, orange, grapefruit, or cranberry)
Soups	Strained cream soups	Broths with chunks, pieces, noodles, or rice
Miscellaneous		Thin beverages such as coffee, tea, water Carbonated beverages

(Consistency: 3 tablespoons instant baby rice to ¾ cup liquid, or commercial thickening agent used according to package directions.)

Thickening Agents

The following readily available products may be used as thickening agents:

- rice cereal
- plain gelatin
- mashed potatoes
- potato flakes
- dry powdered milk
- cornstarch
- plain yogurt

Commercial thickening agents are also available from local pharmacies and through nutrition and speech-language pathology catalogs. Some of the available brands include:

- Thick-it®
- Nutrathick®
- Thick and Easy®
- Thick Set®
- Thixx®
- Frutex®

Guidelines for Selecting Food Consistencies

The following examples and indications can help determine appropriate food consistencies but are general guidelines only. Food consistencies must be individualized for each patient in accordance with the team's recommendations.

Consistency	Examples	Indications
Thick liquids	Thickened, strained soups	**Severe, moderately-severe dysphagia** Impaired mastication, cricopharyngeal dysfunction, reduced pharyngeal peristalsis, reduced oral transit, bolus control
Dysphagia pureed	Smooth cooked cereals, pureed eggs, pudding, pureed strained meat	**Moderate, mild-to-moderate dysphagia** Reduced oral transit, delayed swallow reflex, impaired mastication, reduced pharyngeal peristalsis
Dysphagia advanced pureed	Pureed meat or ground, pureed vegetables, pureed fruits or soft, moist fruit such as banana	**Mild-moderate, mild dysphagia** Vertical chewing, mild-moderate impairments in oral or pharyngeal functioning
Dysphagia mechanical/soft	Soft-cooked fruits, vegetables, ground meat with gravy, cottage cheese, dry cereals which become soft in milk	**Mild dysphagia** Mild deficits in oral transit, decreased rotary chewing, minimal to mild deficits in pharyngeal functioning, poor dental status
Mechanical soft	Ground chopped meat with gravy, canned fruits, soft-cooked vegetables, bread without crust	**Minimal dysphagia** Mildly reduced rotary chewing, other areas normal or minimally impaired

Level 1 Dysphagia Diet: Thickened Liquids

This meal plan provides approximately 1,750 calories, 57 grams of protein, and at least 75 percent of USRDA guidelines for essential vitamins and minerals.

Sample Meal Plan

Breakfast

> 4 oz. pureed strained fruit, diluted with juice
> (Ratio: 2 parts puree strained fruit to 2 parts juice)
>
> 4 oz. strained thinned cereal
>
> 8 oz. thickened milkshake or instant breakfast

Lunch and dinner

> 4 oz. pureed strained fruit, diluted with juice
> (May substitute tomato juice, thickened with gelatin)
>
> 4 oz. whipped, strained potatoes, thinned with soup or gravy
>
> 8 oz. thickened milk shake, eggnog or instant breakfast

Dysphagia Thickened Liquids Diet

	Recommended	Not allowed

Milk products	Whipped cream
	Thickened eggnog
	Thickened instant breakfast
	Thick milk shake
	  (consistency of soft-serve
	  ice cream)
		Ice cream
		Sherbet
		Yogurt

Soups	Thickened, strained soups	Broth, soup with chunk pieces, noodles
Vegetables	Tomato juice, thickened if necessary	Pureed vegetables
Fruits	Pureed strained fruit (diluted with juice)	Undiluted pureed fruit
Potatoes	Whipped, strained potatoes in soup or thinned with gravy	All other potatoes, rice, pasta
Cereal	Strained, thinned with milk	Cold cereal
Fats	Butter, margarine, sour cream mixed with recommended foods	
Miscellaneous	Salt, powdered seasoning, sugar, jelly	Other spices or seasonings

(Consistency: ½ instant baby rice cereal to ½ liquid, less than that of applesauce, or a commercial thickening agent)

Recipes

Strained, Thinned Cereal (makes 2 servings)

4 oz cooked enriched cereal (¾ cup)

1½ Tbsp (4 tsp) margarine

2 Tbsp sugar (if allowed)

3 oz milk (¼ cup)

Melt margarine in hot cereal. Add sugar and mix. Add milk. Blend until very fine. Strain through large mesh strainer.

Thickened Milk Shake or Instant Breakfast

1. Sprinkle 2 Tbsp unflavored gelatin over 1/4 cup cold milk. Stir until completely dissolved. Add 6 more ounces of milk, then mix with appropriate quantity of milk shake mix or instant breakfast mix. Mix thoroughly.

2. Mix appropriate quantity of milk shake or instant breakfast mix with 8 oz milk. Add 3 Tbsp instant baby rice cereal and mix well.

Note: Use high-calorie, high-protein milk shake or eggnog mix which provides at least 260 calories and 15 grams protein per 8 oz. serving and at least 25 percent of the USRDA guidelines for essential vitamins and minerals.

Whipped, Strained Potatoes (makes 2 servings)

½ cup prepared mashed potatoes

1½ Tbsp (4 tsp) margarine

½ cup whole milk, diluted cream soup, or evaporated milk

Melt margarine in mashed potatoes. Add milk or cream soup. Blend thoroughly.

Fortified Pudding

Prepare any flavor of instant pudding following package instructions, using fortified milk. If fortified milk is not allowed, use prepared milk shake to mix with instant pudding.

Fortified Milk (makes 2 cups)

⅔ cup dry skim milk powder

2 cups whole milk

Mix well.

Yogurt Shake (Lee 1981)

¼ cup yogurt

¼ cup ice cream

½ cup gelatin (jelled)

Provides 4 gm protein, 140 calories

Cottage Cheese Shake (Lee 1981)

¼ cup cottage cheese

¼ cup ice cream

½ cup gelatin (jelled)

Provides 8 gm protein, 180 calories

Level 2 Dysphagia Diet: Pureed Foods

This diet is used for a patient who receives nothing by mouth but this diet. All foods must be the consistency of pudding or applesauce. The speech-language pathologist or occupational therapist will request additional foods as the patient demonstrates the ability to tolerate them.

The volume of food is kept very small—most patients can swallow only a few spoonfuls at first, and the goal is to have them focus on their accomplishments, not to feel discouraged by the large volume of food they were unable to eat.

As patients at this stage are often unable to swallow liquids of normal consistency, it is extremely difficult to maintain hydration through oral intake. In some cases the patient's fluid needs must be met by non-oral fluids.

This sample meal plan will provide approximately 1,500 calories, 70 grams of protein, and at least 65 percent of the USRDA guidelines for essential vitamins and minerals. *It does not provide adequate fluids.* Only liquids approved for the individual patient, as determined by the team, are allowed.

Sample Meal Plan

Breakfast
1 egg, pureed
4 oz hot cereal with 1 Tbsp margarine
4 oz pureed fruit

Lunch and dinner
4 oz pureed meat
4 oz pureed vegetable
4 oz whipped potatoes with 1 Tbsp margarine
4 oz fortified pudding

Dysphagia Pureed Diet

	Recommended	Not allowed
Milk products	Pudding, smooth custard, smooth yogurt	Textured pudding, ice cream or yogurt with seeds, skin or pulp
Soups	Thickened, strained soups (with pureed vegetables, meats)	
Meat/poultry/ fish/eggs	Pureed, strained meat Souffle	Eggs, all other meats
Vegetables	Strained, pureed vegetables	Whole, fresh, ground vegetables
Fruits	Strained, pureed fruits	All other fruits, whole, canned or fresh

Dysphagia Pureed Diet
(continued)

	Recommended	*Not allowed*
Potatoes	Smooth, whipped with gravy	All other potatoes, rice, noodles
Cereals	Smooth, cooked cereals (oatmeal, cream of wheat, etc.)	Cold cereal
Fats	Butter, margarine, sour cream	All others
Miscellaneous	Salt, powdered seasonings, sugar, jelly	All others

Note: Only liquids approved for the individual patient as determined by the team are allowed.

Level 3 Dysphagia Diet: Advanced Purees

This diet meets the 1989 USRDA guidelines for essential vitamins and minerals. It provides approximately 2,000 calories and 90 grams of protein. Since many patients at this level have difficulty with oral intake of liquids, the diet provides only 600-700 cc of available fluids.

Sample Meal Plan

Breakfast

- 1 egg, pureed
- 4 oz hot cereal with 1 Tbsp margarine
- 4 oz nectar or juice thickened with pureed fruit
- 4 oz thickened milk shake or instant breakfast

Lunch and dinner

- 4 oz pureed meat
- 4 oz pureed vegetable
- 4 oz whipped potatoes with 1 Tbsp margarine
- 4 oz fortified pudding
- 4 oz thickened milk shake, yogurt shake, or cottage cheese shake

Dysphagia Advanced Pureed Diet

	Recommended	Not allowed
Milk products	Pudding, custard, thick milk shake, yogurt, yogurt shake, cottage cheese shake	Yogurt with seeds, pulp, skin. Thin milk products.
Meat/poultry/ fish/eggs	Pureed meat, pureed meat and pasta casserole, souffle, pureed eggs, cottage cheese or ricotta cheese, pureed meat salads without pickle or vegetable	All other meats, cheese
Vegetables	Pureed vegetables	Whole, fresh or ground
Fruits	Pureed fruit, mashed banana, applesauce	All other fruit, whole, canned or fresh
Potatoes	Whipped	All other potatoes, rice, noodles
Breads	Soft bread without crust or seeds. Pancakes soaked in syrup.	All others
Cereal	Cooked cereals (oatmeal, creamed wheat, creamed rice, etc.)	Cold cereals
Fats	Margarine, butter, sour cream, gravy	All others
Soups	Pureed soups, thickened as necessary	Any soup with chunks of vegetable, starch, or meat. Avoid cream soups if milk products are discontinued.
Miscellaneous	Sugar and jelly may be added to allowed foods	All others

Note: Only liquids approved for individual patient, as determined by the team, are allowed.

Level 4 Dysphagia Diet: Mechanical Soft Foods

This diet meets the 1989 USRDA guidelines for essential vitamins and minerals. It provides 75-100 grams protein and 1,900-2,300 calories. The diet provides 1,000-1,250 cc of available fluid.

Sample Meal Plan

Breakfast
  1 egg, soft-scrambled or hard-poached
  6 oz cooked cereal with 1 Tbsp margarine, and sugar if desired
  Bread with margarine and jelly *or* pancake with margarine and syrup
  4 oz thickened juice
  4-8 oz thickened milk shake

Lunch and dinner
> 2-3 oz ground meat with gravy (very moist)
> ¼-½ cup soft-cooked buttered potato, pasta, rice, or starchy vegetable
> (no corn or legumes)
> ¼-½ cup soft, buttered vegetable
> Bread (crust removed)
> Margarine
> Soft dessert (pudding, ice cream, soft cake, gelatin, soft fruit)
> 4-8 oz thickened juice
> 4-8 oz thickened milkshake

Dysphagia Mechanical Soft Diet

	Recommended	*Not allowed*
Milk products	Pudding, custard, thick milk shakes, yogurt with finely diced fruit, soft-serve ice cream. Cottage cheese, ricotta cheese, ground cheese (as in pimento cheese sandwich filling), melted cheese (in casseroles, souffles)	Thin milk products, yogurt with seeds, skin. Slices or chunks of cheese.
Meat/poultry/ fish/eggs	Ground meat with gravy. Ground meat in casseroles or stews. Finely ground meat salad without pickles or vegetables. Soft sandwiches, no crust. Scrambled, poached, or soft-cooked eggs. Hard-cooked eggs finely ground and mixed with mayonnaise as egg salad. Fish, flaked or mashed, then moistened.	Whole or sliced meats, chunks of meat, fish, poultry, or eggs
Vegetables	Soft-cooked green beans, carrots, beets, spinach, squash (mashed), cauliflower, asparagus (tips only), any pureed vegetable.	Vegetables with tough skins or hard seeds. Legumes. Raw vegetables.
Fruits	Softly cooked apples, peaches, and pears, with skin removed. Mashed ripe banana. Small bites very ripe mashed cantaloupe and watermelon with seeds removed. Pureed fruits.	
Potatoes and starches	Mashed, boiled, baked without skin, scalloped. Rice, noodles, or pasta in cream sauce or casseroles.	

Dysphagia Mechanical Soft Diet
(continued)

	Recommended	Not allowed
Breads and cereals	Soft bread without seeds. Toast (may be softened in coffee or hot chocolate). Dry cereals, such as corn flakes, which become soft in milk. Soft crackers (such as graham crackers, or saltines or vanilla wafers moistened with milk).	Hard rolls, seeded breads. Breads with nuts or raisins. Coarse breads, fried breads. Dry cereals with fruit or nuts, coarse cereals. Seeded crackers.
Desserts	Plain cookies (may be softened in milk or coffee). Plain cake with plain frosting. Cream pie, no crust. Plain doughnut. Soft fruit cobbler (no skins). Soft bread pudding, rice pudding without raisins. Firm gelatin. Cheesecake.	Cookies with nuts, coconut, chocolate chips, or dried fruit. Desserts with berries, seeds, nuts, coconut, dried fruits.
Soups	Pureed soups. Soups without chunks of vegetables or meat.	Soups with chunks of vegetables or meat, dried beans, or peas Cream soups if milk is not allowed.
Fats	Margarine, butter, sour cream, gravy	Other fats
Miscellaneous	Mayonnaise, catsup, mustard, cinnamon, salt and pepper, non-dairy creamers, creamy peanut butter, jelly, syrup, honey	Other condiments. Chunky peanut butter, jams, preserves.

Note: Only liquids approved for individual patient, as determined by the team, are allowed.

Level 5 Dysphagia Diet: Mechanical Soft to Modified General

This diet ranges from a modified mechanical soft to a modified general diet. It allows some flexibility in texture of the foods, but still includes thickened liquids for those patients who remain unable to safely drink thinner liquids.

The texture of the meat should start as ground meat with gravy or ground meat in casseroles or stews. As the patient progresses in ability to chew and swallow, the entree may be finely diced or chopped meat in a meat salad or sandwich filling, or whole-curd cottage cheese.

The crust should be cut off bread. All vegetables should be cooked soft and served moist.

This diet plan meets the 1989 USRDA guidelines for essential vitamins and minerals. It provides approximately 2,000 calories and at least 85 grams of protein.

Sample Meal Plan

Breakfast

1 egg, soft-scrambled or hard-poached

6 oz cooked cereal with margarine and sugar (if desired)

1 slice toast with margarine and jelly

4 oz juice thickened with pureed fruit

8 oz thickened milkshake

Lunch and dinner

3 oz ground (to chopped) meat with gravy

4 oz buttered potato, rice, or pasta

4 oz buttered soft-cooked vegetable

1 slice bread with margarine

4 oz fruit cobbler, cake, custard or fruit

4-8 oz thickened milk shake

4-8 oz thickened juice

or

8 oz casserole with soft meat or cheese and a starch

Mechanical Soft to Modified General Diet

	Recommended	Not Allowed
Milk products	Pudding, custard, thick milk shakes, yogurt with finely diced fruit, sherbet, ice cream.	Thin milk products. Yogurt with seeds, skin.
	Cottage cheese, ricotta cheese, ground cheese (as in pimento cheese sandwich filling). Melted cheese (in casseroles, souffles).	Slices or chunks of cheese
Meat/poultry/ fish/eggs	Ground meat with gravy, progressing to chopped meat with gravy. Ground meat in casseroles or stews. Meat loaf, ham loaf. Finely ground meat salad. Soft sandwiches, no crust. Scrambled, poached, or soft-cooked eggs. Hard-cooked eggs finely ground and mixed with mayonnaise as egg salad. Fish baked or broiled, salmon loaf or tuna croquettes (baked).	Whole or sliced meats, chunks of meat, fish, poultry or eggs
Vegetables	All soft-cooked vegetables	Raw vegetables

Mechanical Soft to Modified General Diet
(continued)

	Recommended	Not Allowed
Fruits	Softly cooked fruits without skin. Canned fruits. Ripe banana. Small bites of very ripe mashed cantaloupe and watermelon with seeds removed	Other raw fruits
Breads and cereals	Soft bread without seeds. Toast (may be softened in coffee or hot chocolate). Dry cereals without dried fruit or nuts. Soft crackers (graham crackers, or saltines or vanilla wafers moistened with milk).	Hard rolls, seeded breads, breads with nuts or raisins. Coarse breads, fried breads. Dry cereals with fruit or nuts, coarse cereals, seeded crackers
Desserts	Plain cookies (may be softened in milk or coffee). Plain cake with plain frosting. Cream pie, no crust. Plain doughnut. Soft fruit cobbler (no skins). Soft bread pudding, rice pudding without raisins. Gelatin. Cheesecake.	Cookies with nuts, coconut, chocolate chips, or dried fruit Desserts with berries, seeds, nuts, coconut, dried fruits
Soups	Pureed soups, cream soups, soups with softly cooked vegetables or meat, noodles, rice or pasta	Plain broth. Cream soups if milk is not allowed.
Fats	Margarine, butter, sour cream, gravy	Other fats
Miscellaneous	Mayonnaise, catsup, mustard, cinnamon, salt and pepper. Non-dairy creamers. Creamy peanut butter, jelly, syrup, honey.	Other condiments. Chunky peanut butter. Jams, preserves.

Note: Only liquids approved for individual patient, as determined by the team, are allowed.

Additional Recipe Sources

Drink to Your Health
Denise LeBlanc Wolford, RN, DNS
8817 Arbor Park
Dallas, Texas 75243

*Dysphagia and Its Management:
A Review for Dieticians*
Kathryn A. Lee, RD
112 Circle Road
Staten Island, New York 10304

Cliffdale Farms
Julio E. Limantour,
Director of Marketing
Route 29, Box 69
Palm, Pennsylvania 18070
   (a good source of gourmet foods developed for consistency-modified diets that can be prepared in medical facilities)

5 ■ Dysphagia Concerns for Speech-Language Pathology

Introduction

Treatment for dysphagia should be based on the knowledge and data derived from the diagnostic swallowing evaluation, and information obtained from videofluoroscopic and manometric studies, where available, as well as from assessments by other team members.

The speech-language pathologist who works with the adult with dysphagia plays a key role in the following management considerations:

- assessing potential for oral intake

- determining method of oral intake

- selecting diet consistency

- specifying risk precautions

- determining candidacy for therapeutic intervention (see Prognostic Considerations, Appendix B, page 103).

- choosing treatment techniques

- suggesting treatment strategies with related professionals

(American Speech-Language-Hearing Association 1990; Cherney et al. 1986)

From the swallowing evaluation, assessment by other team members, and with the above-stated management considerations in mind, the speech-language pathologist establishes long-term goals and short-term goals and provides indirect and direct treatment for swallowing disorders. Specific guidelines follow. Many of the guidelines for treatment have been adapted, with additions and modifications, from Jeri Logemann's 1983 book entitled *Evaluation and Treatment of Swallowing Disorders*.

Setting Goals

Long-Term Goals

Use the Functional Severity Levels for Dysphagia (see Chapter 3, pages 39 to 40) for assistance in developing long-term, functional goals.

Factors to be considered when writing a long-term goal include the following: nutritional intake method (oral, non-oral), diet consistency, quantity and nutritional adequacy of diet, assistance or supervision required, and use of facilitating or compensatory strategies. Samples of long-term goals follow.

- *Safe, nutritionally adequate, oral intake of prescribed puree diet with independent consistent use of facilitating swallowing and feeding strategies.*

- *Safe, nutritionally adequate oral intake of thick liquid diet, with food presented by trained nursing staff or family members using recommended swallowing/feeding techniques.*

Short-Term Goals

Use the Speech-Language Pathology Swallowing Evaluation form (see Chapter 3, page 45) for assistance in developing appropriate, practical short-term goals.

Short-term goals should be written to consider:

- specific, treatable areas of impairment

- the needs of the patient in the immediate future

- functional targets with functional benefits

- the determination of whether treatment will be **indirect**—not involving the introduction of food or liquids by mouth—or **direct.**

Short-term goals involving indirect swallowing therapy include:

- *Improved oral and laryngeal strength, range of motion, and speed.*

- *Improved speed, strength, and consistency of swallow reflex with thermal stimulation 5 times per day.*

Short-term goals which directly involve the use of food and/or liquids and the use of facilitating strategies include:

- *Consistent lip closure during swallow to prevent escape of food or liquid from lips.*

- *Consistent use of facilitating chin flex strategy during liquid by mouth intake with minimal cuing.*

Indirect Treatments

The following treatment exercises do not involve the introduction of food or liquid by mouth. For that reason, they are called *indirect*.

Labial (Lip) Exercises

These exercises are helpful for the patient who has difficulty with lip closure or with holding a straw with the lips. Have patient:

1. Stretch the lips in /i/ position (eee). Hold 1 second.
2. Pucker lips tightly in /u/ position (oo). Hold 1 second.
3. Bring lips together horizontally in /m/ position. Hold 1 second.
4. Hold a straw with the lips only.
5. Hold a tongue depressor between the lips.
6. Hold a small piece of paper between the lips.

Gradually increase time on each of the above tasks, up to 30 seconds. Repeat series 10 times per day. If patient is unable to achieve closure, try closure around a spoon first.

Mandibular (Jaw) Exercises

These exercises are used with the patient who has reduced mandibular strength, range of motion, and difficulty chewing. Have patient:

1. Open jaw as wide as possible. Hold 1 second. Do 5 times.
2. Move jaw to each side as far as possible. Hold 1 second. Do 5 times.
3. Move jaw in a circular fashion. Do 5 times.

Repeat series 10 times per day.

Lingual (Tongue) Exercises

These exercises are used with patients who have difficulty with lingual control of bolus, reduced anterior-to-posterior lingual movement, or incomplete tongue-to-palate contact. Have patient:

1. Open mouth as wide as possible. Elevate (lift) tongue as high as possible in the front, hold 1 second, release. Do this 5 times.
2. Elevate back of tongue as far as possible, hold 1 second, release. Do 5 times with lips parted slightly.
3. Slide tongue to left as far as possible; hold 5 seconds. Do this 5 times.
4. Slide tongue to right as far as possible; hold 5 seconds. Do this 5 times.
5. Slide tongue left to right 10 times.
6. Slide tongue out as far as possible, hold 1 second then pull in. Do this 5 times.
7. Pull tongue in as far as possible, hold 1 second then release. Repeat 5 times.

Do this series of exercises 5 to 10 times each day.

Tongue Thrust Treatment

These exercises are designed to reduce tongue thrust, which can interfere with oral transit. The clinician should:

1. Heighten the patient's awareness of the tongue thrust by providing visual feedback.

2. Ask the patient to consciously position the tongue on the alveolar ridge and do a dry swallow, with an upward-backward push.

3. Use vibration at the temporomandibular joint to discourage thrusting (McCracken 1978).

4. Dab sweet solutions (such as rose-hip syrup) to the sides of the tongue to encourage retraction (Langley 1987, p. 61).

5. Apply pressure to the anterior third of the tongue with tongue blade in a downward and posterior fashion.

Buccal (Cheek) Exercises

These exercises are useful with the patient who pockets food or who has reduced sensitivity in the buccal cavity. Have patient:

1. Round lips tightly and say "oh."

2. Stretch lips laterally and say "ee."

3. Alternate movements for 1 and 2 above, saying "oh [→] ee, oh [→] ee."

4. Smile widely and hold 1 second.

Repeat series 10 times per day.

Resistance and Bolus Control Exercises

These exercises are designed to improve lingual strength and oral control of the bolus. Have patient:

1. Push tongue against tongue blade. Hold for 1 second.

2. Manipulate blade according to clinician's instructions (such as *hold it between tongue and palate,* or *move it side to side*). Verbalize where the blade is and how successful attempts to manipulate are.

3. Move stick of licorice or ring-shaped hard candy (tied to string) in circular fashion in mouth.

If patient succeeds with the above exercises, try these:

4. Move a ⅓ tsp. paste-consistency bolus around mouth with tongue cupped around it. Expectorate bolus rather than swallow. Check for residue.

5. Vary #4 with slightly larger bolus, then with ⅓ tsp. liquid.

6. For exercise in bolus propulsion, place gauze wad soaked in juice in mouth, push upward and backward with tongue, squeezing liquid out (clinician holds gauze).

Soft Palate Exercises

These treatment exercises are used with the patient who has difficulty with velar elevation or with closing off the velopharyngeal port. The exercises are particularly useful for patients who experience nasal regurgitation. The clinician should:

1. Ask patient to produce /ae/ and /a/ alternately with mouth open wide (Langley 1987, p. 61).

2. Stretch patient's tongue by grasping tongue tip in gauze or cotton glove and pulling it gently forward out of the mouth. This movement spreads to the soft palate (Langley 1987, p. 61).

3. Stimulate patient's velum by stroking near the midline with sterile soft brush, iced cotton swab or laryngeal mirror (Langley 1987).

4. If palatal incompetence is a serious problem, a palatal prosthetic device should be considered.

Stimulation of Gag Reflex

This procedure can be used with those patients who do not have a protective gag reflex.

1. Lightly stroke the posterior tongue, soft palate, uvula, palatoglossal and palatopharyngeal arches with a tongue depressor (Silverman and Elfant 1979).

2. Repeat this procedure several times until a gag reflex is elicited.

3. Repeat the entire procedure several times a day.

Note: Many individuals with normal swallowing ability exhibit reduced or absent gag reflexes (DeJong 1967). Currently, there are no data to support the importance of a gag reflex as an indicator of a patient's ability to swallow (Logemann 1983), although it can function as an important mechanism against aspiration and the swallowing of foreign or noxious stimuli.

Laryngeal Adduction Exercises

These exercises facilitate improved laryngeal closure for the patient who has difficulty with airway protection.

Have patient do each of the following exercises 5 to 10 times daily, for 5 minutes each time.

1. While sitting in chair, hold breath tightly and push (or pull) on chair with both hands for 5 seconds.

2. Do same as #1 but with one hand pushing (or pulling), and produce clear voice "AH."

3. Produce "AH" 5 times with hard glottal attack.

4. Produce "AH" with hard glottal attack. Prolong it for 5 seconds.

Producing Productive Cough

These activities can be used with patients who have difficulty producing an effective protective cough. If the patient is being treated for respiratory difficulties, the respiratory or physical therapist will also be working towards effective volitional cough.

1. Encourage the patient to cough whenever needed to clear the airway. Positively reinforce coughing.

2. Place finger and thumb on thyroid and ask patient to cough (Langley 1987, p. 63).

Training the Patient in Supraglottic Swallow

(prior to introducing any liquid or food by mouth)

This technique is a safe swallow strategy for those patients who have difficulty with airway protection. Have patient:

1. Take a small breath and hold it.

2. Pretend to place food or liquid in mouth.

3. Tilt head forward and swallow.

4. Cough immediately after swallow.

5. Swallow again.

Note: Some patients may benefit from repeating steps 4 and 5 after entire sequence (cough after swallow and swallow again).

Stimulating the Swallowing Reflex

This indirect-treatment technique is used with those patients who have a delayed or absent swallowing reflex.

1. Trigger the reflex with a small, long-handled laryngeal mirror (#00, ½″ diameter).

2. Hold the mirror in ice for 10 seconds.

3. Lightly touch it to the base of the anterior faucial arch.

4. Repeat this contact 5 to 10 times. This heightens the sensitivity of the reflex.

5. Ask the patient to close mouth and swallow after stimulation is applied.

6. Repeat this triggering of the reflex 4 to 5 times per day, for 5 minutes each time.

Other Swallowing-Stimulation Techniques

1. Apply a wrapped ice cube to the sternal notch during attempted swallows.

2. Stroke gently upward under the patient's chin.

3. Manually vibrate the laryngopharyngeal musculature, starting under the chin and going down the sides of the larynx.

4. Apply stretch pressure to pharyngeal constrictor muscles with the heels of the hands (from behind) to the base of the skull in a forward and upward fashion.

(Silverman and Elfant 1979)

Direct Treatments

The following direct treatments and facilitating strategies involve the introduction of food or liquid by mouth. They can be done with a therapeutic meal tray or at mealtimes with the patient's regular tray.

Oral, Oral Preparatory Phase

1. Place food on stronger side of oral cavity.
2. Place food on midline of tongue.
3. Apply pressure against cheek, weakened side.
4. Encourage lip closure during chewing and/or swallowing.

If patient exhibits tongue thrust, position food posteriorly on the tongue in an attempt to avoid the thrusting pattern. Also, encourage an upward-backward push to begin the swallow. One way to encourage this push is to apply firm, downward, posterior pressure with spoon.

Pharyngeal, Velopharyngeal Phase

1. Maintain 90° upright posture.

with pharyngeal peristalsis problems:

2. Alternate liquid vs. solid swallows.
3. Swallow 2 times in succession per bolus.
4. Limit amounts per swallow.

with unilateral pharyngeal paralysis:

5. Turn head to weaker side, or tilt head to stronger side.

with delayed reflex or poor velar functioning:

6. Chin flex down.
7. Limit bolus to ½ to 1 level tsp.
8. Thermal stimulation of swallow reflex (see p. 72).

with reduced laryngeal functioning:

9. Supraglottic swallow (see p. 72).
10. Chin flex down.
11. Clear throat or cough after swallow.
12. Vocalize after swallow; if vocal quality is wet and gurgly, clear throat and swallow again.

Stimulating the Swallowing Reflex

This direct method can be used if the patient can tolerate small amounts of material. Gradually introduce small amounts of liquid following stimulation.

1. Use a straw as a pipette, filled with about ¼″ of ice water.

2. Place the pipette's iced end at the same point where the laryngeal mirror contacted the anterior faucial arch.

3. Ask the patient to swallow when you release the liquid and say "swallow now."

4. For additional stimulation, use limeade or ginger ale instead of ice water.

Once the swallow reflex begins to consistently trigger, gradually increase the amount and consistency of the food presented at the anterior faucial arches.

Supraglottic Swallow

The following describes an actual sequence of the safe swallowing technique when introducing liquid or food by mouth.

1. Take a small breath and hold it.

2. Place food/liquid in mouth.

3. Tilt head forward and swallow.

4. Cough immediately after swallow.

If the patient has been NPO, introduce liquids gradually. Give only ⅓ tsp. of liquid at first—from a teaspoon, not a cup. Gradually increase to ½ tsp. and then 1 tsp. as patient progresses without difficulty.

6 ■ Dysphagia Concerns for Occupational Therapy

Introduction

Occupational therapy for feeding/swallowing disorders involves facilitation of safe, adequate, independent feeding.

First, the occupational therapist gathers information from the feeding evaluations and assessments by other team members concerning:

- body positioning
- upper-extremity range of motion* and incoordination
- physical endurance
- bilateral upper extremity functioning
- unilateral neglect
- sensory deficits
- motor planning deficits
- cognitive deficits
- influence of abnormal reflexes.

The occupational therapist then establishes a treatment plan. The plan includes short- and long-term goals for each aspect of the feeding/swallowing problem. It also includes suggested primary and secondary treatment techniques to increase the patient's level of independence in each problem area. Adaptations and equipment are recommended that will promote improved positioning and independence in self-feeding.

The following specific guidelines are based on a problem-oriented approach. (See Appendix G, page 113, for a list of suppliers of adaptive equipment.)

Body Positioning

Problem

Poor body positioning, secondary to limited head and/or trunk control, and inability to properly position extremities in order to complete self-feeding/ swallowing safely and independently.

Short-Term Goal

To assume an upright posture in a chair with extremities supported and maintain proper positioning during a meal (30 to 45 mins.).

Long-Term Goal

To consistently assume and maintain an upright posture in a chair with proper body positioning for all meals.

Suggested Treatment

Primary: Participate in upper-extremity reaching tasks to increase dynamic sitting balance and protective/ equilibrium reactions.

Secondary: Participate in functional mobility tasks such as bed mobility, transfers, and ambulation during activities of daily living. Participate in sitting or standing activities for increasing time periods.

Adaptations—Methods and Equipment

Pillows, rolled blankets, or towels can assist with positioning in a chair, wheelchair, or bed. Wheelchairs can be adapted to accommodate poor trunk and head control or to provide proper positioning of affected extremities. Adaptations include head supports, lateral trunk supports, lapboards, back and seat inserts, arm/leg supports, and other body-positioning devices*.

Comments

The ideal eating position is to be as upright as possible with hips bent at 90 degrees. The head should be held in body midline and tilted slightly forward with the chin tucked.

Poor body positioning may result in possible choking and aspiration. If there is extremity paralysis, the affected extremities must be adequately positioned to prevent pain or any interference during the feeding/swallowing process. Being comfortable and able to enjoy a meal encourages independence. It is important to keep positioning adaptations as simple as possible since it may be difficult for family and staff to consistently maintain proper positioning of these adaptations.

Upper Extremity Range of Motion/Incoordination

Problem

Limitations in upper-extremity range of motion and/or incoordination preventing self-feeding.

Short-Term Goals

- To increase upper-extremity range of motion in order to effectively complete self-feeding using appropriate adaptive methods/equipment.
- To increase upper-extremity coordination in order to use a functional grasp/release and hand-to-mouth pattern for self-feeding.

Long-Term Goal

To complete self-feeding as independently as possible using adaptive methods and equipment as needed in order to use a functional grasp/release and hand-to-mouth pattern.

Primary: Provide passive and active range of motion to upper extremities. Engage in activities specifically focusing on increasing joint movement. Promote upper-extremity coordination through use of gross and fine motor tasks that develop an active grasp/release and movements that encourage a functional hand-to-mouth pattern. During mealtime, give hands-on assistance to promote effective hand-to-mouth pattern and grasping of utensils.

Secondary: Teach compensatory methods of grasp/release and use of a functional hand-to-mouth pattern. Teach use of adaptive equipment to compensate for inability to maintain a functional grasp. Provide specialized splints to increase passive range of motion or functional grasping. Promote effective ways to stabilize the upper extremities during self-feeding.

Adaptations—Methods and Equipment

Forks, spoons, and knives with various styles and sizes of built-up handles are used for easier grasping and more effective manipulation of the utensils.

Extension handles on forks and spoons compensate for limited shoulder motion. Curved or bent handles and swivel-type utensils compensate for limited forearm rotation and wrist motion. Sporks* of various types limit the number of utensils needed for self-feeding.

Universal cuffs* of many styles compensate for inability to maintain an effective grasp during self-feeding. There are many types of splints available to hold eating utensils and to compensate for poor wrist/forearm control. Various specialized splints* may be used to promote a functional hand position for self-feeding (such as air splints, volar or dorsal resting hand splints, wrist cock-up splints, and dynamic splints that encourage active movements).

Weighted utensils, cups, cup holders, or cups with lids compensate for incoordination problems such as tremors or ataxic movements of upper extremities and trunk. Long straws or straw holders can compensate for poor trunk control or limited forward trunk motion. Place mats made of Dycem® or other brands of nonskid material can prevent a plate or bowl from moving around. A wet cloth can also stabilize a plate or bowl.

An inner-lip plate, scoop dish/bowl, or plate guard can enable the patient to more effectively place food onto a fork or spoon (Glickstein et al. 1989, pp. 5-6). Various types of arm supports compensate for limited active range of motion and/or decreased upper extremity strength during feeding. Some examples of upper-extremity supports* include: ball bearing feeders, table clamp arm positioners, arm troughs with swivel, offset suspension feeders, and adapted feeding harnesses (Takai 1986, pp. 420-424).

Comments

Finger feeding may be easier than using utensils. Using a lapboard or resting the elbows on a table can help stabilize the upper extremities.

It is important to keep adaptive equipment simple. It is also important to acknowledge when a patient is unwilling to accept an adaptive device—even when it promotes functional independence.

Physical Endurance

Problem

Inability to tolerate self-feeding or swallowing for entire meal secondary to limited physical endurance.

Short-Term Goal

To easily tolerate self-feeding and effectively swallow throughout a portion of a meal.

Long-Term Goal

To easily tolerate self-feeding and effectively swallow throughout an entire meal.

Suggested Treatment

Primary: Have patient participate in various gross motor activities to develop physical endurance (such as standing while completing an upper-extremity task at shoulder height or moving to various work stations to complete different manipulative tasks at shoulder height). To increase dynamic sitting endurance, have patient engage in an upper-extremity task at shoulder height. To increase rate and effectiveness of swallow, have client participate in swallowing activities.

Secondary: Have patient participate in self-care, leisure, or home-management tasks, gradually increasing the amount of time he or she is engaged in the task. Teach energy conservation techniques to be used during a meal (such as take a bite of food, place utensil down and rest between bites). Teach relaxation techniques focusing on deep breathing in order to promote energy conservation.

Adaptations—Methods/Equipment

Provide physical assistance as patient reaches his or her maximal level of physical endurance.

Comments

It is important to recognize the patient's physical limitations for his or her safety. To have several mini-meals with small portions can promote feeding/swallowing independence and increase physical endurance at the same time.

Bilateral Upper-Extremity Function

Problem

Inability to functionally use both upper extremities in order to effectively complete two-handed self-feeding tasks.

Short-Term Goals

- To effectively use adaptive methods/equipment in order to successfully use a knife for spreading/cutting.
- To effectively use one hand for self-feeding.

Long-Term Goal

To effectively self-feed using one hand and adaptive methods/equipment as needed.

Suggested Treatment

Primary: Provide opportunities to learn one-handed eating techniques using adaptive methods and equipment as appropriate. Train patient to effectively use nondominant hand. Provide opportunity to manipulate various adaptive devices for self-feeding.

Secondary: Participate in a variety of one-handed tasks that increase patient's fine and gross motor skills.

Adaptations—Methods and Equipment

A variety of adaptive devices are available to compensate for use of one hand for self-feeding and meal preparation. A rocker knife is used to cut food with one hand by using a rocking motion. An inner-lip plate can assist with scooping food onto a utensil instead of using two hands. For meal preparation, a cutting board with nails or a board with a small lip can enable the patient to slice food or spread food onto a slice of bread (Glickstein et al. 1989, p. 6.)

Comments

Providing as many opportunities as possible to practice one-handed techniques will help the patient succeed with self-feeding. One-handed techniques also help the patient become independent in meal preparation and other activities of daily living.

Unilateral Neglect

Problem

Inability to consistently locate food items on the plate or tray when items are positioned on the affected side of the body.

Short-Term Goal

To consistently locate food items on the plate/tray 50 percent of the meal with occasional verbal/visual cuing.

Long-Term Goal

To consistently locate food items on the plate/tray throughout entire meal with occasional verbal/visual cuing.

Suggested Treatments

Primary: Provide activities that reinforce awareness of the affected side of the body. Use mini-meals to reinforce consistency in looking at the entire plate/tray. Have client name aloud the various items on the plate/tray (ask client to point to an item, name it, take a bite or sip of the item, and then name the item again).

Secondary: Have patient participate in a variety of self-care, home management, and leisure activities that give successful opportunities to look to the affected side of the body.

Adaptations—Methods/Equipment

Teach compensatory techniques (such as turning the plate around so the food is always within visual range) to patient/family/staff. Position other items on the tray within visual range. Use auditory cuing to draw attention to the affected side. Use a mirror to provide the patient with visual reinforcement of swallowing effectiveness (Glickstein et al. 1989, p. 8.)

Comments

Unilateral neglect can occur as a result of a deficit in the central processing system of the right parietal lobe. Learning compensatory techniques for this type of problem is more difficult and often less successful than with other visual perceptual disturbances (Trombly and Scott 1978, p. 111).

Sensory Deficits

Problem 1: Pocketing

Consistently pockets food on the affected side and is unable to clear food from affected side of mouth.

Short-Term Goal

To consistently clear food from affected side of mouth with verbal cuing and to chew majority of food on unaffected side of mouth.

Long-Term Goal

To consistently clear food from affected side of mouth and chew majority of food on unaffected side.

Suggested Treatments

Primary: Provide sensory stimulation techniques to increase tactile sensitivity to affected side of mouth.

Sensory stimulation techniques include, but are not limited to, the following techniques:

- olfactory stimulation which is associated with the discrimination of four tastes (salt, sweet, sour, and bitter) (Langley 1987, p. 31)
- brushing to increase sensitivity to light touch (Stockmeyer 1967, p. 937)
- applying vibration to the central muscle mass for up to 3 minutes to increase proprioceptive awareness (Langley 1987, p. 57). Deep pressure to inhibit the tactile defensive reactions (Ayres 1980, p. 110).

Secondary: Train patient/family/staff in sensory stimulation techniques to be done prior to eating.

Problem 2: Locating Food

Unable to locate food items on plate/tray on hemianopic* side.

Short-Term Goal

To consistently locate food items on plate/tray on hemianopic side with verbal cuing.

Long-Term Goal

To consistently locate food items on plate/tray on hemianopic side.

Suggested Treatments

Primary: Provide activities which require looking to hemianopic side in order to complete the task (such as a table-top eye-hand coordination activity). Use mini-meals to provide successful experiences with locating food on plate or tray. Give verbal/tactile/gestural cuing as needed; decrease amount of cuing as patient becomes more successful and independent.

Secondary: Encourage participation in simple self-care activities (such as dressing or simple home-management tasks—picking up clothes around the bedroom). Provide leisure-time activities that promote increased awareness of hemianopic side (such as reading, board games, crafts, and plant care).

Adaptations—Methods and Equipment

Teach compensatory techniques for loss of sensation in the mouth (such as using unaffected hand to help clear the mouth). Use a mirror to encourage increased visual awareness of the hemianopic side and to be more aware of pocketing food. Use fingertips of unaffected hand to assist in locating food on the plate or tray. Position food in a specific pattern on the plate and put other items in consistent positions on the tray.

Comments

It is important to use an intact sensory system when teaching compensatory techniques for visual and tactile deficits. Patients whose perceptual deficits are coupled with sensory losses will have greater difficulty learning compensatory techniques (Trombly and Scott 1978, p. 117).

Sensory input is needed to trigger the swallow reflex. Salivation can provide sensory input and is stimulated by taste, texture, temperature, pressure, and olfactory stimulation (Silverman and Elfant 1979, pp. 384-385). Lemon-glycerine swabs and flavored ice pops will provide sensory stimulation to the oral cavity. Beef broth and other oily liquids will thin secretions; milk-based products will thicken secretions (Silverman and Elfant 1979, pp. 384-385).

It is important to have good mouth and dental/denture care before and after feeding. A clean oral cavity will prevent infection and promote salivation.

Motor Planning Deficits—Apraxia

Problem

Inability to consistently complete hand-to-mouth pattern and inappropriate use of utensils during meals.

Short-Term Goals

- To consistently complete hand-to-mouth pattern with minimal physical assistance during a meal.
- To consistently use utensils appropriately throughout a meal with verbal and tactile cuing provided.

Long-Term Goals

- To consistently complete hand-to-mouth pattern with occasional verbal cuing in order to complete a meal.
- To consistently use utensils appropriately during a meal with occasional verbal cuing needed.

Suggested Treatment

Primary: Encourage tactile-kinesthetic input to both upper extremities. Prior to self-feeding, promote weight-bearing activities to the extremity being used for eating. Use a hand-over-hand method to guide the upper extremity through the hand-to-mouth pattern, and then have the patient immediately repeat the pattern without physical guidance. Provide verbal, visual, and tactile cuing as needed during a meal in order to consistently manipulate the utensil correctly.

Secondary: Provide activities to experience the hand-to-mouth pattern (such as picking up objects to look at closely or to smell or taste).

Adaptations—Methods/Equipment

Provide verbal, written, or gestural cuing prior to using physical assistance. Use a backward chaining method to teach the hand-to-mouth sequence. This will provide frequent repetition of the pattern and promote independence.

Comments

There are many types of apraxia*. The two types that may affect self-feeding and swallowing abilities are *ideomotor apraxia* and *ideational apraxia*. Ideomotor apraxia refers to difficulty completing a motion on command, though the motion may be completed at an automatic level. Ideational apraxia—the inability to execute the act automatically—is more limiting (Trombly and Scott 1978, p. 112). The prognosis for relearning a feeding skill when apraxia is a primary problem is limited, particularly when cognitive deficits are also present.

Cognitive Deficits

Problems

- Inability to consistently use good safety techniques during self-feeding/swallowing.
- Inability to attend to self-feeding in order to complete a meal.
- Inability to remember appropriate eating/swallowing methods in order to complete a meal.

Short-Term Goals

- To consistently use good safety techniques throughout self-feeding/swallowing with verbal, visual, and tactile cuing.
- To consistently attend to self-feeding with verbal, visual, and tactile cuing.
- To consistently remember appropriate eating/swallowing methods with verbal, visual, and tactile cuing in order to complete a meal.

Long-Term Goals

- To consistently use good safety techniques throughout self-feeding/swallowing with occasional verbal cuing.

- To consistently attend to self-feeding with occasional verbal cuing.
- To consistently remember appropriate eating/swallowing methods with occasional verbal cuing.

Suggested Treatment

Primary: Use mini-meals to provide opportunities to decrease impulsiveness, increase attention to specific aspects of self-feeding/swallowing, and to teach appropriate techniques for safe, independent self-feeding/swallowing. Give verbal/visual cuing to redirect patient.

Secondary: Engage in different types of activities that will increase attention span, ability to concentrate on a specific aspect of a task, and improve short-term memory.

Adaptations—Methods and Equipment

- Provide an environment free of visual/auditory distractions.
- Provide opportunities to talk about the meal and the important aspects of using good safety techniques.
- Provide consistency in a daily schedule and in following a specific routine associated with feeding.

Comments

Cognitive deficits that affect self-feeding/swallowing may require constant supervision. The patient may achieve maximal independence in a small-group situation. Being a part of a small group may increase the patient's ability to focus on the meal (by observing others in the group). Small-group membership can also help with other important aspects of self-feeding/swallowing.

Abnormal Oral Reflexes

Problem 1: Bite Reflex

Reflex interferes with placement of food in mouth and removal of utensil.

Short-Term Goal

To minimize the influence of the bite reflex during presentation of food into the mouth and to avoid eliciting the bite reflex.

Long-Term Goal

To effectively place food and eating utensils in the mouth without the bite reflex interfering.

Suggested Treatment

Primary: Properly position body, with head upright and chin slightly tucked, in order to minimize the influence of a bite reflex. Apply pressure to the temporomandibular joint, thrusting the jaw forward to open mouth. Never pry mouth open or pull utensils out of mouth. Wait for mouth to open spontaneously, and encourage opening with verbal directions (*Open your mouth*) (Groher 1984, p. 140).

Secondary: Brush lateral part of teeth and gums with soft toothbrush positioned between teeth and cheeks (Silverman and Elfant 1979, p. 390). Stimulation of the masseter muscles should be avoided if a bite reflex exists (Groher 1984, p. 140).

Problem 2: Suck-Swallow Reflex

Reflex interferes with smooth intake of food secondary to the inability to voluntarily break the suck-swallow pattern.

Short-Term Goal

To functionally use a voluntary suck-swallow pattern for smooth food intake.

Long-Term Goal

To have smooth food intake without the influence of abnormal suck-swallow reflex.

Suggested Treatment

Primary: Present the straw. Allow patient to consume a safe amount of liquid bolus (1 or 2 sips), then withdraw the straw. Reintroduce the straw and repeat the procedure. Teach patient the above technique to minimize the influence of suck-swallow during oral intake. Place a gloved finger in corner of lips to break suction of lips around the straw (Silverman and Elfant 1979, p. 391).

Secondary: Present lollipop or ice pop; allow patient to suck-swallow 2 or 3 times then withdraw stimulus. Encourage patient to concentrate on breaking the pattern; provide physical assistance as needed to break the pattern (Groher 1984, p. 140).

Repeat the above exercise to increase voluntary control of the suck-swallow. Apply pressure to the tip of the tongue to stimulate automatic sucking (Groher 1984, p. 141).

Comments

Oral reflexes of adults are divided into two categories: *normal* (such as the cough or gag reflex) and *abnormal* (such as the bite, suck-swallow, or tongue thrust) (Groher 1984, p. 138). Inhibition or reduction of abnormal oral reflexes is discussed here. The suck-swallow reflex may be used to promote a reflexive swallow in the initial stages of treatment when a voluntary swallow is absent (Groher 1984, p. 140).

7 ■ Patient Care Information Sheets

Introduction

This chapter contains a number of patient-care forms. The regular use of these forms will help ensure that all personnel involved in caring for the patient are aware of dysphagia-related precautions and procedures.

The forms are all reproducible. They include:

- *ATTENTION! Feeding and Swallowing Instructions*
- *Patient Is NPO*
- *Dysphagia Flow Sheet*
- *Dysphagia Flow Sheet, Page 2: Nursing Progress Notes*
- *Medicine Administration Sheet*
- *Aspiration Precautions for Oral Feeders.*

Using the *ATTENTION!* Sheet

The *ATTENTION!* sheet is used to tell all staff and visitors about the patient's swallowing disorder as it relates to diet, positioning, and the patient's needs during the feeding/swallowing process.

The sheet is filled out by the speech-language pathologist and occupational therapist and is placed on the bulletin board beside the patient's bed. The multidisciplinary swallowing team updates the *ATTENTION!* sheet as the patient progresses.

To complete the *ATTENTION!* sheet:

1. Highlight the appropriate "Dysphagia Level Description." Check the liquids that the patient can safely tolerate, as appropriate.

2. Check the items in the "Positioning" section that facilitate improved oral feeding. Selected items are to be determined by examinations by the speech-language pathologist and the occupational therapist.

3. Check the appropriate supervision and required level of assistance in the "Patient Needs" section. Also check facilitating swallowing strategies according to the results of the speech-language pathologist's swallowing evaluation.

4. List any appropriate adaptive equipment, as recommended by the occupational therapist.

5. Add any additional comments (such as *check oral cavity after meal for residue*) needed to ensure the patient's safety and success during the feeding/swallowing process.

Using the *Patient Is NPO* Sheet

The charge nurse fills out the *Patient Is NPO* sheet and places it on the patient's door as soon as it is determined that the patient cannot safely take any food or liquid by mouth.

The sheet is removed when the patient's feeding/swallowing abilities have improved enough that it is safe to have food or liquid by mouth. The NPO status is changed only after a speech-language pathology/occupational therapy evaluation and consultation with physician.

Write the patient's name in the space provided; enter the date and nurse's signature at the bottom of the sheet.

Using the *Dysphagia Flow Sheet*

The *Dysphagia Flow Sheet* documents the specific progress of the patient as he or she progresses from non-oral feeding through various levels of oral feeding. The sheet is used by the staff member working with the patient and is completed at the end of the meal.

The *Dysphagia Flow Sheet* covers seven days and includes three meals daily. To initiate the use of the sheet, the speech-language pathologist or occupational therapist completes the patient identification information and adds the sheet to the nursing section of the patient's chart. A new sheet is started each week or with each change in diet consistency.

Staff members who supervise or assist with each meal initial the appropriate box of each section of the flow sheet for each meal.

The dietitian highlights two days each week when a specific calorie count sheet will be filled out (see Appendix I, page 117). This sheet is completed by the staff member supervising or assisting at mealtime and is analyzed by the dietitian.

Specific Instructions

Tolerates swallowing. Note whether any difficulties occur during swallowing (such as coughing, choking or spitting out).

Consistency not tolerated. Document the food or liquid consistency presented at that mealtime that the patient has difficulty managing.

Level of responsiveness. Note how alert and cooperative the patient is at that particular meal and indicate how well the patient responds to physical or verbal assistance during the meal.

Intake. Document the percentage of food eaten and amount, expressed in cc's of liquid consumed (see page 2 of the flow sheet for a list of normal volume values). Use the top portion of the square to document milk consumed and the bottom half to document juices consumed.

Physical assistance given. Report the amount of physical assistance the patient required during a meal in order to complete the feeding/swallowing process successfully and safely. Check *maximal* when it was necessary for the feeding aide to physically intervene in 8 out of 10 attempts to complete the feeding/swallowing process. Use *moderate, minimal,* and *slight* when lesser degrees of assistance are needed. *None* indicates that no physical intervention was necessary in order for the patient to eat safely and successfully.

Verbal assistance given. Note the amount of verbal assistance necessary during a meal in order for the patient to eat safely and successfully. Use the same guidelines as for physical assistance.

Amount of time. Indicate how much time the patient requires to either finish the meal or become unable to continue as a result of being too tired or unsafe. This information helps in setting guidelines for a functional time frame for meal consumption. The severity and type of dysphagia, and the patient's physical endurance and behavior, are key factors in determining how much time it takes the patient to complete the meal.

Page 2: Nursing Progress Notes

Page 2 of the flow sheet provides space for nursing progress notes. Nursing staff should use this space to document any significant changes in the patient's abilities or behavior.

Using the *Medicine Administration Sheet*

The *Medicine Administration Sheet* is filled out by the charge nurse at the initial multidisciplinary swallowing team meeting, or immediately after receiving necessary information from the speech-language pathologist or occupational therapist. The sheet is kept in the medicine administration record.

The *Medicine Administration Sheet* provides nursing staff with the following information. For maximum visibility, the form should be photocopied on yellow paper (or paper of some other bright color not reserved for specialized forms).

Dysphagia severity. This ranges from *severe nonfunctional dysphagia* to *minimal dysphagia.* The severity level is based on findings of the speech-language pathologist's swallowing evaluation.

Dysphagia diet. This indicates the consistency of diet, ranging from thick liquids to mechanical soft.

Fed by. This indicates those trained staff and family members responsible for feeding or supervising the patient at meals.

Medicine administration. This specifies the method of administering medicine consistent with the patient's swallowing ability and diet consistency.

Using the *Aspiration Precautions for Oral Feeders* Sheet

The *Aspiration Precautions for Oral Feeders* sheet is used to inform staff and visitors of a particular patient's need for special precautions at meals and during medicine administration.

It is generally used for those patients who do not, or who no longer, require assistance with specific feeding or swallowing strategies (as indicated on the *ATTENTION!* sheet).

The sheet should be displayed on the bulletin board beside the patient's bed.

ATTENTION!

Feeding and Swallowing Instructions

_____ in room # _____

as dysphagia, a swallowing disorder. Patient has difficulty swallowing safely and should be given only items
eat or drink on the following prescribed diet.

Dysphagia Level	Description	Comments
0	NPO Suction available Diagnostic trial feeding by dysphagia team ST/OT	
1	Thick liquids Suction available	
2	Dysphagia pureed diet with: ☐ thick ☐ medium ☐ thin liquids	
3	Dysphagia advanced pureed diet with: ☐ thick ☐ medium ☐ thin liquids	
4	Dysphagia mechanical soft diet with: ☐ thick ☐ medium ☐ thin liquids	
5	Mechanical soft diet with: ☐ thick ☐ medium ☐ thin liquids	

When patient is fed, please observe the following instructions for patient safety:

Positioning

☐ 90 degrees upright from hips
☐ chin flexed down
☐ support neck with pillows

☐ elevate weaker arm
☐ up for 30 min. after feeding
☐ turn head to weaker, paralyzed side
          left   right

Patient needs

☐ 1:1 supervision/assist by nursing
☐ close supervision/restorative feeding
☐ place food on stronger side of mouth
☐ place food on middle of the tongue
☐ alternate liquids with solid swallows
☐ use spoon only

☐ thermal stimulation
☐ straw
☐ take small bites, ½ to 1 level tsp.
☐ verbal reminder to swallow
☐ to cough or clear throat and say "ah"
☐ check inside mouth for pocketing

Adaptive equipment used _____

_____

Other comments_____

_____

Date:_____   Dysphagia team leader: _____

Patient Is NPO

For medical or safety reasons,

this patient _____, Room No. _____

Is

NPO

Not to receive anything to eat or drink by mouth

Please do not give this patient anything to eat or drink.

Please check with charge nurse if you have any questions.

Thank you

Nurse _____

Date _____

Dysphagia Flow Sheet

name _____ Patient no. _____ Room no. _____

TOLERATES SWALLOWING	B	L	D	B	L	D	B	L	D	B	L	D	B	L	D	B	L	D	B	L	D
Refused																					
Unable																					
Choking/strangling																					
ing out/some choking																					
Coughing after																					
Without difficulty																					
NSISTENCY *NOT* TOLERATED																					
Thick liquids																					
Dysphagia pureed																					
Dysphagia advanced																					
Mechanical soft																					
Thin/medium liquids																					
LEVEL OF ESPONSIVENESS																					
Poor																					
Fair																					
Good																					
INTAKE																					
Food %																					
Milk (liq. oz.)																					
Juice (liq. oz.)																					
SICAL ASSISTANCE GIVEN																					
Maximal: 8-10/10																					
Moderate: 6-7/10																					
Minimal: 4-5/10																					
Slight: 1-3/10																					
None: 0/10																					
RBAL ASSISTANCE GIVEN																					
Maximal: 8-10/10																					
Moderate: 6-7/10																					
Minimal: 4-5/10																					
Slight: 1-3/10																					
None: 0/10																					
MOUNT OF TIME																					
45-60 minutes																					
30-45 minutes																					
15-30 minutes																					
0-15 minutes																					

ur initials in the appropriate boxes for *each* section. Write comments on the back as needed.

_____ Multidisciplinary swallowing team member: _____

ommunication Skill Builders, Inc./602-323-7500
ay be reproduced for administrative use. (Catalog No. 7807)

Dysphagia Flow Sheet
Page 2: Nursing Progress Notes

Family name _____ First name _____

Attending physician _____ Room no. _____ Hosp. no. ___

Date	Time	Nurses' Progress Notes

Normal values: Large glass—240cc; Juice glass—120cc; Plastic-foam cup—180cc; Soup bowl (large)—240cc; S (small)—180cc; 1/2 pint milk—240cc; Ice cream—120cc; Insulated mug—210cc ; China cup—180cc; Coffee bottle—300c carafe—300cc; Water carafe—960cc; Water cup—120cc.

Medicine Administration Sheet

Name_____

Dysphagia severity_____

Dysphagia diet _____

Fed by _____

See *ATTENTION!* sheet
(posted at bedside and in nursing section of chart)
for additional information.

Medicine administration
(check appropriate block)

☐ Crush med

☐ Administer with applesauce

☐ Liquid meds only

☐ NPO

☐ Special instructions _____

_____

_____

Must have 1:1 supervision by trained dysphagia staff

- -

Medicine Administration Sheet

Name_____

Dysphagia severity_____

Dysphagia diet _____

Fed by _____

See *ATTENTION!* sheet
(posted at bedside and in nursing section of chart)
for additional information.

Medicine administration
(check appropriate block)

☐ Crush med

☐ Administer with applesauce

☐ Liquid meds only

☐ NPO

☐ Special instructions _____

_____

_____

Must have 1:1 supervision by trained dysphagia staff

- -

Medicine Administration Sheet

Name_____

Dysphagia severity_____

Dysphagia diet _____

Fed by _____

See *ATTENTION!* sheet
(posted at bedside and in nursing section of chart)
for additional information.

Medicine administration
(check appropriate block)

☐ Crush med

☐ Administer with applesauce

☐ Liquid meds only

☐ NPO

☐ Special instructions _____

_____

Must have 1:1 supervision by trained dysphagia staff

- -

Aspiration Precautions

for

Oral Feeders

1. Elevate head of bed 90 degrees at mealtime and during oral administration of medication. Support upper back/shoulders/neck with a pillow.

2. Visually check the mouth for pocketing of food in cheeks.

3. Provide mouth care every 4 hours.

4. Do not lower head of bed to less than 45 degrees for at least 30 minutes after eating.

5. Watch closely during meals and when administering medicine.

Glossary

Achalasia. Failure of muscles to relax. Achalasia of the cardia occurs when the cardiac sphincter fails to relax, resulting in difficulty of passage of foods to the stomach. Dysphagia may be severe in advanced cases.

Apraxia. The inability to execute a volitional, purposeful act in the absence of sensory or other motor deficits.

Aspiration. The action of material penetrating the larynx and entering the trachea below the level of the vocal folds.

Basal energy expenditure (BEE). An estimate of a patient's baseline caloric requirements using the patient's height, weight, age, and sex. Actual kilocalorie requirements are then estimated by multiplying the BEE by a factor which accounts for the activity level and stress of illness.

Body positioning devices

adult foam torso support: Used for patients who slump forward in wheelchairs. Has adjustable straps.

arm sling: Provides support for an arm. The type of sling chosen will depend on the specific problems of the dysphagic patient and should be determined by an occupational or physical therapist.

knee spreader. Widens the sitting base through increased hip abduction to provide seat support.

padded head support. Designed to fit high-backed wheelchairs of any width with adjustable sides.

posture guard. A trunk support system with adjustable straps. Provides a constant stabilizing force against the body. Securely attaches to back of wheelchair.

seat cushion. Provides increased support of the hips and lower extremities.

wheelchair arm tray kits. Provide various types of support of an arm. The base is a sturdy plastic arm tray which secures to the wheelchair armrest. The arm can be supported on dense foam in an elevated position, on the plastic tray or on a cloth.

Bolus. Food or liquid placed in the mouth for ingestion.

Cricopharyngeal myotomy. Surgical procedure involving external incision through the side of the neck into the cricopharyngeal muscle, slitting it from top to bottom to divide and open the sphincter. Used with patients who have cricopharyngeal dysfunction.

Enteral feeding. A non-oral feeding that makes use of any portion of the gastrointestinal tract.

Hemianopic. Loss of vision in half the visual field in one or both eyes.

Hydration. Balance of electrolytes and fluid in body.

Nosey cut-out cup. Adaptive cup with cutout space for nose. Used with persons who have difficulty tipping head back or extending the neck. Sometimes used to deter a patient who has poor airway protection or delayed swallow from tipping head back when drinking.

NPO. An instruction (*non per oral*) used to indicate that the patient should not receive any food, liquid, or medicine by mouth.

Pyriform sinus. A space formed between fibers of the interior constrictor muscle and the sides of the thyroid cartilage.

Range of motion

    active: To move a joint through its full range of movement with assistance from the patient.

    passive: To move a joint through its full range of movement without any assistance from patient.

Reflux. Abnormal movement of stomach contents back up into the esophagus.

Scintigraphy. Dynamic imaging technique that permits detection and quantification of bolus flow, transit times, and percentage of aspiration.

Splints

    Various devices used to promote function and prevent contractures/deformities of the extremity to which the splint is applied.

    air splint: a pliable double sheeting of plastic that holds a limb in a specified position. Air pumped into the splint provides sufficient pressure to maintain an appropriate limb position.

    dorsal splint: a splint applied to the backside of the arm.

    dynamic splint: a splint that has movable components which enable an extremity to move, increasing range of motion and muscle strength.

    volar splint: a splint applied to the palm or side of the arm.

    wrist cock-up splint: a splint applied to the arm in order to position the wrist in extension.

Spork. A combination of a spoon and fork. Has the bowl component of the spoon with modified fork tines.

Suctioning. A method for removing excessive secretions or food from the airway. May be applied to the oral, nasopharyngeal, or tracheal passage.

Universal cuff. A strap that is secured around the hand with a small pocket in which utensils may be placed. The universal cuff holds utensils when a patient cannot maintain an effective grasp on various utensils.

Upper extremity supports

> **arm trough with swivel:** an arm trough which can be used with the ball bearing feeder, the table clamp arm positioner, or the offset suspension feeder. It provides greater elbow flexion and extension and supports the forearm in an appropriate position.

> **ball bearing feeder:** Helps patients with poor to fair deltoid power perform self-feeding and various other functional activities. Designed for persons with severe shoulder girdle weakness. Feeder supports the weight of the arm; ball bearings allow easier movement. Elevating proximal arm models use rubber bands to assist lifting, shoulder abduction, and elbow flexion or extension.

> **offset suspension feeder:** can be attached to the wheelchair or a movable frame. Supports the upper extremity in an anti-gravity position. Rotation occurs at the side of the arm at the ball bearing joint. Straps and arm supports are adjustable to increase arm movement.

> **table clamp arm positioners:** positioners for persons with shoulder girth weakness who do not use a wheelchair. An arm positioner is attached to a table or desk by a sturdy clamp.

Valleculae. A wedge-shaped space between the base of the tongue and the epiglottis.

Videofluoroscopic swallowing study. A radiographic study, often referred to as a *modified barium swallow,* used to define etiology of aspiration, assess oral and pharyngeal transit times, pinpoint motility difficulties, and examine vocal cord closure. The evaluation utilizes three consistencies (liquid, paste, solid) laced with barium.

Web. A membrane or tissue that crosses a space; an esophageal web extends across the esophageal lumen and impairs swallowing.

References

American Speech-Language-Hearing Association (ASHA). 1990. Knowledge and skills needed by speech-language pathologists providing services to dysphagic patients/clients. *ASHA Supplement* 32:7-8.

Ayres, J. A. 1980. *Sensory integration and the child.* Los Angeles: Western Psychological Services.

Bach, D., S. Pouget, K. Bell, M. Kilfoil, M. Alfiere, J. McEnvoy, and G. Jackson. 1989. An integrated team approach to the management of patients with oropharyngeal dysphagia. *Journal of Allied Health.* Fall:459-68.

Bass, N. H. 1988. Neurogenic dysphagia: Diagnostic assessment and rehabilitation of feeding disorders in the neurologically impaired. *Advances in Clinical Rehabilitation* 2:186-228.

Bonanno, P. 1971. Swallowing dysfunction after tracheostomy. *Annals of Surgery* 174(1): 29-33.

Cameron, J. L., J. Reynolds, and G. D. Zuidema. 1973. Aspiration in patients with tracheostomies. *Surgery, Gynecology, and Obstetrics* 136:68-70.

Castell, D. O., and M. U. Donner. 1987. Evaluation of dysphagia: A careful history is crucial. *Dysphagia* 2:65-71.

Cherney, L., C. Cantieri, and J. Pannell. 1986. *Clinical evaluation of dysphagia.* Rockville, MD: Aspen Systems Corporation.

DeJong, R. 1967. *The neurologic examination.* New York: Hoeber Medical Division, Harper and Row.

Ehrlich, A. B. 1970. *Training therapists for tongue thrust correction.* Springfield, IL: Charles C. Thomas.

Ekedahl, C., I. Mansson, and N. Sandberg. 1974. Swallowing dysfunction in the brain-damaged with drooling. *Acta-Otolaryngologica* 78:141-49.

Emick-Herring, B., and P. Wood. 1990. A team approach to neurologically based swallowing disorders. *Rehabilitation Nursing* 15:126-32.

Erlichman, M. 1989. The role of speech-language pathologists in the management of dysphagia. Washington, DC: Department of Health and Human Services, Publication no. 89-3437.

Farber, S. D. 1982. *Neurorehabilitation: A multi-sensory approach.* Philadelphia: W.B. Saunders.

Feldman, R., K. Kapur, J. Alman, and H. Chauncy. 1980. Aging and mastication changes in performance and the swallowing threshold with natural dentition. *American Geriatrics Society* 28:97-103.

Fleming, S. 1984. Treatment of mechanical swallowing disorders. In *Dysphagia: Diagnosis and management,* edited by M. E. Groher. Stoneham, MA: Butterworth Publishers.

Fleming, S., R. Nelson, J. Muz, and S. Hamlet. 1989. Scintigraphy in the dysphagic patient. Paper presented to the American Speech-Language Hearing Association, St. Louis, MO.

Glickstein, J., D. Olson, L. Cherney, and E. Pollard. 1989. Feeding and swallowing problems in the elderly: An interdisciplinary approach. *Focus on Geriatric Care and Rehabilitation* 2:1-8.

Griffin, K. 1974. Swallowing training for dysphagic patients. *Archives of Physical Medicine and Rehabilitation* 55:467-70.

Groher, M. E. 1984. *Dysphagia diagnosis and management.* Stoneham, MA: Butterworth Publishers.

Guymer, A. J. 1986. Handling the patient with speech and swallowing problems. *Physiotherapy* 72:276-279.

Hillhaven dietary manual for long-term care facilities. 1991. Tacoma, WA: Hillhaven Corp.

Hulme, J. B., J. Shaver, S. Archer, and C. E. Mullette. 1987. Effects of adaptive seating devices on the eating and drinking of children with multiple handicaps. *American Journal of Occupational Therapy* 41:81-89.

Jordan, K. 1979. Rehabilitation of the patient with dysphagia. *Ear, Nose, and Throat Journal* 58:59-61.

Kasprisin, A., H. Clumeck, and M. Nino-Murcia. 1989. The efficacy of rehabilitative management of dysphagia. *Dysphagia* 4:48-52.

Kirschner, H. S. 1989. Causes of neurogenic dysphagia. *Dysphagia* 3:184-88.

Langley, J. 1987. *Working with swallowing disorders.* Oxon, England: Winslow Press.

Lee, K. 1981. *Dysphagia and its management: A review for dietitians.* (Available from K. A. Lee, 112 Circle Road, Staten Island, N.Y. 10304)

Lieberman, A. N., L. Horowitz, P. Tedmond, L. Pachter, I. Lieberman, and M. Liebowitz. 1980. Dysphagia in Parkinson's disease. *American Journal of Gastroenterology* 74:157-60.

Logemann, J. 1983. *Evaluation and treatment of swallowing disorders.* San Diego, CA: College Hill Press.

Logemann, J., G. Sisson, and R. Wheeler. 1980. The team approach to rehabilitation of surgically treated oral cancer patients. *Proceedings of the National Forum on Cancer Rehabilitation* 222-27.

Malamud, I. G. 1986. Nutritional support and the occupational therapist's role. *American Journal of Occupational Therapy* 40:343-46.

Mansson, I., and N. Sandberg. 1975. Oro-pharyngeal sensitivity and elicitation of swallowing in man. *Acta-Otolaryngologica* 79:140-45.

Marshall, J. B. 1985. Dysphagia, pathophysiology, causes, and evaluation. *Postgraduate Medicine* 77:58-68.

McCracken, A. 1978. Drool control and tongue-thrust therapy for the mentally retarded. *American Journal of Occupational Therapy* 32:79-85.

Miller, R. M., and M. E. Groher. 1990. *Medical speech pathology.* Rockville, MD: Aspen Publishers, Inc.

Mueller, H. A. 1972. Facilitating feeding and prespeech. *Physical therapy services in the developmental disabilities.* P. H. Pearson and C. E. William, eds. Springfield, IL: Thomas.

Nash, M. 1988. Swallowing problems in the tracheotomized patient. *Otolaryngologic Clinics of North America* 21:701-09.

Newman, P., and C. Medina. 1987. Dysphagia: A transdisciplinary approach. *Occupational Therapy Forum.* March 18:7-9.

Ogg, H. L. 1975. Oral-pharyngeal development and evaluation. *Physical Therapy* 55:235-41.

Ottenbacher, K., A. Bundy, and M. A. Short. 1983. The development and treatment of oral-motor dysfunction: A review of clinical research. *Physical Therapy and Occupational Therapy in Pediatrics* 3:147-60.

Ottenbacher, K., T. Hicks, A. Roark, and J. Swinea. 1983. Oral sensory-motor therapy in the developmentally disabled: A multiple baselines study. *American Journal of Occupational Therapy* 37:147-60.

Ottenbacher, K., B. S. Dauck, V. Grahn, M. Gevelinger, and C. Hassett. 1985. Reliability of the behavioral assessment scale of oral function in feeding. *American Journal of Occupational Therapy* 3:147-60.

Ray, S. A., A. C. Bundy, and D. L. Nelson. 1983. Decreasing drooling through techniques to facilitate mouth closure. *American Journal of Occupational Therapy* 37:749-53.

Royal, V. et al. 1987. Written communication as reported in *The role of speech-language pathologists in the management of dysphagia.* Washington, DC: Department of Health and Human Services. Publication No. 89-3437:5.

Roueche, J. R. 1980. *Dysphagia: An assessment and management program for the adult.* Minneapolis: Sister Kenny Institute.

Rusk Institute of Rehabilitation Medicine. 1984. *Protocol for team management for patients with dysphagia.* New York: New York University Medical Center.

Sammons, F. 1990. Fred Sammons Catalog. P.O. Box 32, Brookfield, IL.

Sauerland, E. K., and N. Mizuno. 1970. A protective mechanism for the tongue: Suppression of genioglossal activity induced by stimulation of trigeminal proprioceptive afferents. *Experientia* 26:1226-1227.

Schultz, A., P. Niemtzow, S. Jacobs, and F. Naso. 1979. Dysphagia associated with cricopharyngeal dysfunction. *Archives of Physical Medicine and Rehabilitation* 60:381-86.

Silverman, E. H., and I. L. Elfant. 1979. Dysphagia: An elevation and treatment program for the adult. *American Journal of Occupational Therapy* 33:382-92.

Steefel, J. 1981. *Dysphagia rehabilitation for neurologically impaired adults.* Springfield, IL: Charles C. Thomas.

Stockmeyer, S. A. 1967. An interpretation of the approach of food to the treatment of neuromuscular dysfunction. *American Journal of Physical Medicine* 46:900-56.

Stratton, M. 1981. Behavioral assessment scale of oral functions in feeding. *American Journal of Occupational Therapy* 35:719-21.

Takai, V. L. 1986. The development of a feeding harness for an ALS patient. *American Journal of Occupational Therapy* 40:420-24.

Tesman, B., and B. Michela. 1970. The stroke team concept as implemented in the area III regional medical program. *Stroke* 1:19-22.

Trombly, C., and A. Scott. 1978. *Occupational therapy for physical dysfunction.* Baltimore: Williams and Wilkins.

Trott, M. C., and A. D. Maechtlen. 1986. The use of overcorrection as a means to control drooling. *American Journal of Occupational Therapy* 40:701-04.

Weiss-Lambrou, R., S. Teteault, and J. Dudley. 1989. The relationship between oral sensation and drooling in persons with cerebral palsy. *American Journal of Occupational Therapy* 43:155-61.

Werbowetzki, C. L. 1989. Dysphagia from start to finish: A clinical approach to diagnosis and treatment of the dysphagic patient. Paper presented at conference by Progressive Physical Therapy, Inc., and Med Therapy Rehabilitation Services, Raleigh, NC.

Appendixes

Letter to the Family of the Adult with Dysphagia

Dear family member:

Welcome to our facility's multidisciplinary swallowing team program.

As you know, swallowing is difficult for your family member. Your family member has a condition known as *dysphagia*.

Dysphagia appears in many forms. Mild dysphagia often makes it difficult to manage water and other thin liquids. People who have the most severe forms of dysphagia may not be able to swallow without significant risk of *aspiration*—drawing food or other material into the airway.

Aspiration is dangerous; it can cause choking and may lead to infection. In some cases, alternate means of maintaining nutrition must be used with people who have severe dysphagia.

Our team program has two basic goals. The first goal is to make sure your family member receives safe, adequate nutrition. Adequate nutrition is a vital part of maintaining and improving health, strength, and general well-being. The swallowing team will do all it can to make sure your family member receives sufficient nutrition.

The second goal is to help your family member return to normal swallowing and eating whenever possible.

Speedy, vigorous professional care can help your family member recover as quickly and completely as possible. First, the physician and the speech-language pathologist determine the type and severity of dysphagia. Then the full team goes into action.

Here are some of the people who will work with your family member:

- the **physician** plays a leading role in planning feeding procedures and in overall medical management.
- the **nursing staff** is primarily responsible for caring for your family member. Nurses regularly communicate with the physician, monitor intake, weights, nutritional status, and fluid levels, and ensure safety.
- the **dietitian** and the **speech-language pathologist** make sure that proper diet consistencies are provided. The dietitian also determines nutritional needs and level of intake to make sure your family member's diet is adequate.
- the **occupational therapist** determines whether your family member can eat safely without help. If necessary, the occupational therapist will recommend special equipment or positions to make eating safer and easier.
- the speech-language pathologist, occupational therapist, and nursing staff (and often the **physical therapist** or **respiratory therapist**) design and begin a rehabilitation program specially tailored for your family member.

You are a vital part of the team. Your participation, attitudes, and wishes have a direct effect on how well your family member responds to rehabilitation. You should be as involved and informed as possible during each step of the program.

Please get in touch with any member of the multidisciplinary swallowing team if you have any questions.

Sincerely,

_____

for the multidisciplinary swallowing team

Prognostic Considerations

The following points should be taken into consideration when selecting patients with dysphagia for treatment.

- Type of disorder (oral or pharyngeal dysfunction)

- Underlying cause of dysfunction amenable to treatment

- Swallowing videofluoroscopy results that indicate the presence of disorders affecting the oral preparatory, oral, or pharyngeal phase of swallowing and suggest potential benefit from rehabilitative therapy.

- Absence of medical problems that might preclude participation in treatment, such as respiratory distress.

- Level of alertness.

- Ability to follow and remember simple instructions.

- Willingness to participate in treatment.

- Availability of a support system for follow-through.

(Royal, V. et al. 1987)

Appendix C

Knowledge and Skills Needed by Speech-Language Pathologists Providing Services to Dysphagic Patients/Clients

Task Force on Dysphagia American Speech-Language-Hearing Association

The following document, drafted by the American Speech-Language-Hearing Association (ASHA) Task Force on Dysphagia, was adopted as an official statement by the ASHA Legislative Council (LC 25-89) in November 1989. Members of the task force during development of the document were Michelle M. Ferketic, coordinator, 1988-89; Lee Ann Golper, Marion C. Kagel; Patricia G. Larkins, coordinator; and Suzanna E. Morris. Teris K. Schery, vice president for clinical affairs, was monitoring vice president.

Introduction

A position statement was adopted by the Legislative Council in 1986 (LC 19-86) that recognized the role of the speech-language pathologist in providing services to dysphagic individuals. In the report of the Ad Hoc Committee on Dysphagia, it was suggested that in order to provide these services, education in dysphagia had to be acquired, (American Speech-Language-Hearing Association Ad Hoc Committee on Dysphagia 1986); however, the specific proficiencies, knowledge, and skills required to evaluate and treat dysphagic individuals were not outlined. Therefore, the Executive Board of ASHA established a task force on dysphagia to develop a statement describing the knowledge and skills needed by the speech-language pathologist to provide services to dysphagic patients/clients. This statement is not intended to duplicate the Ad Hoc Committee's report; rather it expands upon the suggestions made regarding the development of clinical proficiencies for speech-language pathologists working with dysphagic individuals. The intent of this statement is to present a comprehensive list of roles, range and scope of skills, and knowledge base needed to provide services to this population. Depending upon the individual's work environment and population(s) served, every speech-language pathologist will not necessarily need to develop proficiencies in all roles.

Some roles are clinical and the speech-language pathologist will need to develop proficiencies based upon the populations served (e.g., adult, developmentally delayed, head and neck cancer). Some roles are administrative in nature and would be best performed by a person with longer experience in supervising. Achievement of proficiencies should be documented and systematic plans for attaining proficiency should be in place in settings serving dysphagic individuals.

Key Terms (or) Definitions

Key terms used throughout this statement have been operationally defined below:

- **Dysphagia**—A swallowing disorder. The signs and symptoms of dysphagia may involve the mouth, pharynx, larynx, and/or esophagus.
- **Oral Intake**—Arm and hand coordination required to bring food from plate to mouth. However, in some literature, oral intake is defined as: (a) placement of food in the mouth; (b) oral gestures used to prepare food for the swallow and gain pleasure from eating; and (c) tongue movement to initiate the oral swallow.
- **Stages of Swallow**—Three stages of deglutition or four phases of ingestion have been delineated in classic research: oral preparation, oral, pharyngeal and esophageal. Recent studies indicate that these stages are most clearly distinguished during small bolus swallows. These stages may overlap during large bolus swallows and during natural "non-command" swallows. Other variables as yet undefined may also affect the clear delineation of these phases.
- **Cough**—A brainstem reflex protecting the entrance to the airway from foreign material.
- **Gag**—A brainstem reflex elicited by contact of a foreign stimulus to the back of the tongue, soft palate, or pharynx, resulting in contraction and elevation of the pharynx and larynx to push the stimulus up and out of the pharynx or to prevent entrance to the pharynx. This neuromuscular action is the

---

American-Speech-Language-Hearing Association. 1990. Knowledge and skills needed by speech-language pathologists providing services to dysphagic patients/clients. *Asha* *32* (Suppl. 2) 7-12. © 1990 by American-Speech-Language-Hearing Association. Used with permission.

opposite of the neuromuscular coordination used in swallow. The gag cannot be used to predict the presence or adequacy of a swallow and is not a protective reflex for a swallow.

- **Diagnostic Technique**—A procedure that provides information on the anatomy and physiology of the swallow.
- **Bolus**—The food, liquid, or other material placed in the mouth for ingestion.
- **Aspiration**—Occurs when food/liquid (bolus) penetrates the airway below the true vocal folds (i.e., subglottic). This can occur (a) before the pharyngeal response; (b) during the pharyngeal response; and (c) after the pharyngeal response. Some literature defines aspiration as airway penetration concomitant with inhalation.
- **Laryngeal Penetration**—Occurs when food/liquid penetrates the portion of the airway above the vocal cords (i.e., supraglottic area). This can occur normally and can also occur before, during, or after the pharyngeal response.
- **Treatment Strategy**—A strategy employed to improve swallowing.

Indirect—Strategies that do not employ the use of foods or liquids.

Direct—Strategies that do employ the use of foods or liquids.

Compensations/Facilitations—Strategies that impose alteration in behavior (i.e., posture, rate, learned airway protection maneuvers), bolus characteristics (i.e., volume, method of intake, consistency) to achieve functional swallowing.

- **Functional Swallow**—A swallow which may be abnormal or altered but does not result in aspiration. This type of swallow does not ensure maintenance of adequate nutrition and hydration.
- **Ingestion/Swallow**—Refers to all processes, functions, and acts associated with bolus introduction, preparation, transfer, and transport.
- **Deglutition**—Refers only to acts associated with bolus transfer and transport.
- **Alternate Nutrition Device/Oral Intake System**—Provides hydration and nutrition in cases when the patient with disordered swallow is unable to ingest a sufficient amount orally without risk of medical complications (e.g., Intravenous [IV], Nasogastric Tube [NG], Jejunostomy, Percutaneous Endoscopic Gastrostomy [PEG], Total Parenteral Nutrition [TPN]).
- **Supplemental Nutrition Device/Oral Intake System**—Assists hydration and nutrition needs in cases when a patient/client

can orally ingest without risk of medical complication but is unable to do so consistently secondary to fatigue, appetite disorders, and so forth.
- **Potential Risks**

Professional—Inappropriate or uninformed patient/client management that compromises the life of the patient/client, promotes medical complications, and/or fails to provide acceptable nutritional support.

Patient—Medical complications that result from dysphagia symptomatology and/or inappropriate uninformed patient/client management.

Setting—Inappropriate patient/client care and management with resulting medical complications to the patient/client.

Roles, Proficiencies, Knowledge

The roles, proficiencies, knowledge bases and skills that enable the speech-language pathologist to provide a continuum of services for dysphagic patients/clients appropriate to the population served are described below:

1.0 Role: Identification of Individuals at Risk for Dysphagia.

Proficient In:

1.1 Recognition of signs and symptoms of dysphagia;

1.2 Review of medical status as diagnosed by the patient's/client's physician(s);

1.3 Determination of cognitive, communication, behavioral, and social status;

1.4 Determination of current oral intake situation (e.g., positioning, staffing, noise level) and method; and

1.5 Communication of results and recommendations to management team.

Knowledge Base and/or Skills Needed:

1.a Knowledge of the medical diagnoses, cognitive and linguistic characteristics contributing to dysphagia;

1.b Knowledge of factors in the oral intake situation that may contribute to dysphagia;

1.c Knowledge of oral intake methods (oral and non-oral) and the problems associated with each that may contribute to dysphagia;

1.d Knowledge of signs and symptoms of dysphagia in the patient's/client's behavior, medical history, medical status;

1.e Knowledge of methods for communicating a patient's/client's need for physiologic dysphagia assessment;

1.f Knowledge of physiologic assessment strategies for use with dysphagic patients/clients; and

1.g Skills in interpretation of risk factors for dysphagia.

2.0 Role: Conduct a Clinical Oral-Pharyngeal and Respiratory Examination with a Detailed History.

Proficient In:

2.1 Identification of abnormal structure;

2.2 Identification of abnormal function;

2.3 Identification of significant symptoms, medical conditions, and medications pertinent to dysphagia;

2.4 Interpretation of examination findings; and

2.5 Documentation of examination findings.

Knowledge Base and/or Skills Needed:

2.a Knowledge of normal, oral-pharyngeal, respiratory structure;

2.b Knowledge of normal, oral-pharyngeal, respiratory function;

2.c Knowledge of significance and implications of abnormal findings as they relate to swallowing;

2.d Knowledge of normal swallowing physiology;

2.e Knowledge of medical conditions and signs and symptoms associated with dysphagia;

2.f Knowledge of limitations of the clinical examination, specifically with regard to detecting aspiration;

2.g Knowledge of how to provide documentation that is concise, thorough, objective, and interpretive;

2.h Knowledge of tracheostomy tubes and their effect on pharyngeal, laryngeal, and respiratory functioning;

2.i Knowledge of unique aspects of ventilator dependent patients/clients and respective roles of others during examination of these patients/clients; and

2.j Knowledge of and skills in conducting an oral-pharyngeal respiratory examination and obtaining a thorough history.

3.0 Role: Conduct Instrumental/Structural Physiologic Examination with Related Professionals.

Proficient In:

3.1 Identification of available and appropriate testing resources (e.g., equipment, personnel);

3.2 Recommendation of appropriate instrumentation techniques (e.g., videofluo-roscopy, manometry, electromyography, ultrasonography);

3.3 Utilization of instrumental technique that can be done jointly with a physician;

3.4 Interpretation of information from examination that can be done jointly with physician; and

3.5 Documentation of examination findings with recommendations that can be done jointly with a physician.

Knowledge Base and/or Skills Needed:

3.a Knowledge of all existing instrumental techniques (e.g., videofluoroscopy, manometry, electromyography, ultrasonography) including their advantages and limitations in terms of particular patient/client populations and types of swallowing disorders;

3.b Knowledge of the variability of normal swallowing behaviors (e.g., bolus volume, consistency, age);

3.c Knowledge of variables to be introduced (e.g., posture change, bolus size, maneuvers) during the instrumental assessment(s) to ensure an optimal examination;

3.d Knowledge of and skills in videofluoroscopic studies of deglutition including the identification of disordered anatomy and physiology;

3.e Knowledge of interpretation of the data resulting from these assessments; and

3.f Knowledge of how to provide documentation of the results of the various assessments that is concise, thorough, objective, and interpretive, and involves other professionals as appropriate.

4.0 Role: Determination of Patient/Client Management Decisions Regarding: (a) methods of oral intake; (b) risk precautions; (c) candidacy for intervention; and (d) treatment strategies with Related Professionals.

Proficient In:

4.1 Identification of relevant supportive and personnel services;

4.2 Identification of acceptable oral intake methods;

4.3 Education of supportive personnel;

4.4 Identification of intervention strategies appropriate to patient's/client's medical condition, swallowing disorder, cognitive status, and behavioral status;

4.5 Identification of potential risks and appropriate precautions;

4.6 Documentation of management decisions; and

4.7 Identification of short and long term goals targeting outcomes.

Knowledge Base and/or Skills Needed:

4.a Knowledge of parenteral and enteral non-oral devices/oral intake systems, recommendations, and medical risks;

4.b Knowledge of and skills in identifying precaution procedures designed to reduce medical risks associated with alternate and supplemental oral intake devices/ systems;

4.c Knowledge of and skills in all existing treatment procedures;

4.d Knowledge of advances in treatment procedures and potential application from other fields;

4.e Knowledge of candidacy, intervention procedures criteria and skills in communicating this information;

4.f Knowledge of and skills in identifying supportive personnel and service needs;

4.g Knowledge of and skills in accessing, educating, and utilizing supportive personnel and referral services; and

4.h Knowledge of and skills in establishing team decisions, documentation procedures, and implementation of these procedures.

5.0 Role: Provide Treatment with Related Professionals as Appropriate.

Proficient In:

5.1 Identification of patient's/client's need for diet modification or status of oral intake in provision of all types of treatment;

5.2 Identification of patient's/client's need for direct or indirect treatment as differentiated from mealtime management;

5.3 Interpretation of patient's/client's response to treatment;

5.4 Quantification of patient's/client's response to treatment;

5.5 Communication of patient's/client's progress/status in treatment;

5.6 Revision of treatment when appropriate;

5.7 Identification of patient's/client's need for re-evaluation; and

5.8 Determination of criteria for discharge/dismissal from treatment.

Knowledge Base and/or Skills Needed:

5.a Knowledge of principles and procedures pertaining to learning and behavior modification;

5.b Knowledge of the anatomy and physiology of the patient's/client's swallowing disorder;

5.c Knowledge of the patient's/client's language, cognitive, and behavioral characteristics;

5.d Knowledge of the patient's/client's medical status;

5.e Knowledge of treatment strategies described in the literature including direct and indirect, and all compensatory techniques;

5.f Knowledge of techniques and skills in quantifying change in swallowing performance;

5.g Knowledge of appropriate diet choices at various points in treatment;

5.h Knowledge of the prognosis for conditions causing dysphagia, and their progress in recovery or deterioration; and

5.i Skills in provision of treatment for a variety of swallowing disorders.

6.0 Role: Provide Education, Counseling, and Training to Patient, Family, Significant Others, Dysphagia Team, and Health Professionals.

Proficient In:

6.1 Identification of educational needs;

6.2 Provision of educational programs;

6.3 Development of continuing education programs;

6.4 Provision of counseling regarding swallowing disorders;

6.5 Provision of patient advocacy;

6.6 Instruction of non-speech-language pathology staff in treatment techniques, problem solving, trouble shooting, and monitoring patient/client status;

6.7 Documentation of education, counseling, and training provided; and

6.8 Evaluation of teaching effectiveness.

Knowledge Base and/or Skills Needed:

6.a Knowledge of education principles;

6.b Knowledge of counseling principles;

6.c Knowledge of and skills in adjusting content and delivery to the level of the person being educated, counseled, or trained;

6.d Knowledge of and skills in applying behavior modification principles;

6.e Knowledge of signs indicating risk;

6.f Knowledge of risk intervention possibilities; and

6.g Knowledge of and skills in monitoring patient/client status.

7.0 Role: Manage and/or Participate in Interdisciplinary Dysphagia Team.

Proficient In:

7.1 Identification of core team members and supportive services;

7.2 Facilitation of team communication;

7.3 Maintenance of team focus;

7.4 Documentation of team activity; and

7.5 Appropriate consultation procedures to and from other team members and other services.

Knowledge Base and/or Skills Needed:

7.a Knowledge of the roles and responsibilities of team members in dysphagia management;

7.b Knowledge of the specialized expertise of interdisciplinary team members pertinent to dysphagia evaluation and treatment;

7.c Knowledge of and skills in facilitating and maintaining team communication and interaction;

7.d Knowledge of and skills in team management, goal direction, and service delivery models;

7.e Knowledge of and skills in specialized consultation needs and procedures for referral;

7.f Knowledge of and skills in appropriate methods of documentation that delineate team decisions and recommendations;

7.g Knowledge of data and procedures that administrators need in the interest of supporting a dysphagia team (e.g., cost accounting and productivity factors); and

7.h Knowledge of basic management and administrative procedures.

8.0 Role: Maintain Quality Control/Risk Management Program.

Proficient In:

8.1 Identification of quality indicators (e.g., structure, process, outcomes);

8.2 Systematic monitoring of quality indicators;

8.3 Resolution of identified problems;

8.4 Identification and communication of risk factors to patient/client, family, and team members;

8.5 Utilization of appropriate risk management procedures (e.g., resolution of identified risk factors, routine revision of quality assurance monitors); and

8.6 Documentation of quality assuranc[e] process.

Knowledge Base and/or Skills Needed:

8.a Knowledge of Quality Assurance po[li]cies established by regulatory bodie[s] (e.g., Joint Commission on Accredita tion of Health Organizations);

8.b Knowledge of institution—specific ris[k] management policies and procedures

8.c Knowledge of quality indicators for dys phagia (e.g., structure: gloves are wor[n] when conducting oral-pharyngeal res piratory exams; process: clinical exam inations include specified larynge[al] assessment tasks; outcome: individu als with dysphagia do not develop pu[l] monary complications secondary t[o] direct treatment of dysphagia);

8.d Knowledge of and skills in using meth ods for monitoring indicators;

8.e Knowledge of and skills in resolution [of] identified problems including collabora tive team efforts;

8.f Knowledge of and skills with infectio[n] control procedures;

8.g Knowledge of risks of aspiration;

8.h Knowledge of causes of aspiration;

8.i Knowledge of and skills with ways t[o] prevent aspiration;

8.j Knowledge of speech-language patho[l] ogists' scope of practice and Code [of] Ethics;

8.k Knowledge of and skills with institution specific policies and procedures con cerning liability prevention and liability

8.l Knowledge of and skills with institution specific documentation policies an[d] procedures; and

8.m Knowledge of tracheal obstructio[n] management techniques (e.g., suction ing and Heimlich maneuver).

9.0 Role: Provide Discharge/Dismissal Plannin[g] and Follow-up Care.

Proficient In:

9.1 Identification of discharge/dismissal cr[i] teria;

9.2 Identification of discharge needs for pa tient and family;

9.3 Identification of need for follow-up car[e] including frequency of treatment mon toring and/or re-evaluation; and

9.4 Documentation of discharge criteri[a] discharge plan and follow-up care.

Knowledge Base and/or Skills Needed:

9.a Knowledge of and skills in establishing discharge criteria;

9.b Knowledge of and skills in assessing discharge needs, establishing a team oriented discharge plan, and coordinating services required;

9.c Knowledge of and skills in determining criteria for follow-up care and establishing policies and procedures to meet identified needs;

9.d Knowledge of and skills in appropriate documentation of discharge criteria, discharge plan, and follow-up care; and

9.e Knowledge of and skills in accessing team recommendations pertinent to dysphagia follow-up care and developing procedures for implementation.

10.0 Role: Teach and Supervise Persons, CFY, Supportive Personnel, and Student-in-Training.

Proficient In:

10.1 Identification of education and clinical training needs;

10.2 Education techniques;

10.3 Supervisory skills;

10.4 Documentation of teaching and supervision; and

10.5 Evaluation of teaching effectiveness.

Knowledge Base and/or Skills Needed:

10.a Knowledge of previous coursework and present proficiency of the trainee;

10.b Knowledge of education principles;

10.c Knowledge of supervision principles;

10.d Knowledge of and skills with requisite documentation;

10.e Knowledge of and skills with methods of evaluating trainee performance; and

10.f Skills in providing effective teaching and supervision.

11.0 Role: Provide Public Education and Advocacy for Serving Individuals with Dysphagia.

Proficient In:

11.1 Provision of methods for public education and advocacy regarding the needs of dysphagic patients/clients;

11.2 Provision of testimony to various governmental, regulatory, and educational agencies; and

11.3 Provision of assistance in obtaining funding for services from appropriate sources.

Knowledge Base and/or Skills Needed:

11.a Knowledge of funding sources and intermediary services provisions pertinent to dysphagia;

11.b Knowledge of advocacy, legal, and regulatory procedures that affect the needs of dysphagic individuals;

11.c Knowledge of public education sources and procedures for increasing awareness of special need groups;

11.d Knowledge of available education aids designed to assist pertinent education and advocacy positions; and

11.e Skills in public education or advocacy.

12.0 Role: Conduct Research.

Proficient In:

12.1 Review and interpretation of existing and pertinent literature;

12.2 Selection of appropriate research design and methodology;

12.3 Interpretation of findings; and

12.4 Dissemination of research findings.

Knowledge Base and/or Skills Needed:

12.a Knowledge of existing literature in normal swallow and dysphagia. Skills in obtaining and interpreting this literature;

12.b Knowledge of and skills in applying research design;

12.c Knowledge of and skills in data collection techniques on normal and abnormal swallow and their advantages and limitations;

12.d Knowledge of and skills in data reduction techniques for each data collection strategy;

12.e Knowledge of and skills in procedures for statistical analyses and their advantages and limitations; and

12.f Knowledge of and skills in scientific writing and dissemination of research findings.

References

American Speech-Language-Hearing Association. Ad Hoc Committee on Dysphagia. 1988. Ad Hoc Committee on Dysphagia Report *Asha* 29:57-58.

American Speech-Language-Hearing Association. 1988. Code of Ethics of the American Speech-Language-Hearing Association. *Asha* 30:47-48.

Instructions to "Feel For" the Swallow

During the swallow the caregiver places his or her fingers under the patient's chin with fingers placed as shown on the diagram below.

1. Place index finger immediately behind mandible, anteriorly. This placement enables the examiner to assess initiation of tongue movement.
2. Place middle finger on the hyoid bone to perceive hyoid bone movement.
3. Place the third finger at the top of the thyroid cartilage. This position and the following position aid in the assessment of laryngeal movement and initiation of the swallowing reflex.
4. Place the fourth finger at the bottom of the thyroid cartilage.

(Logeman 1983, pp. 120-121)

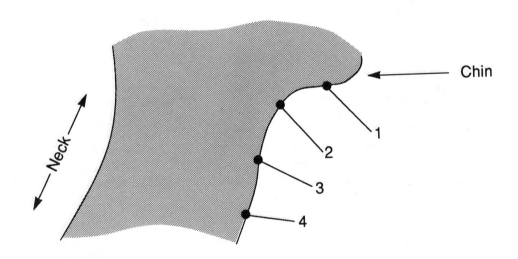

Appendix E

Supervised Feeding Groups

The following section describes possible feeding groups available to the graduate of the multidisciplinary swallowing program, for those patients in rehabilitation or extended care facilities. Five levels of eating are suggested.

The highest-functioning feeding level is for primarily independent feeders. Four patients sit at a table and receive assistance only if needed to cut meat, butter bread, or open milk cartons. These patients are able to manage utensils independently, use appropriate table manners and are essentially independent in functional mobility within the facility.

The assisted feeding group is the next level. This group includes patients who require more verbal encouragement than physical assistance to complete a meal.

Members of this group may not demonstrate socially acceptable mealtime behavior. They do, however, respond well to social situations and benefit from increased socialization. This type of feeding group usually needs setup help such as:

- opening cartons/packets
- cutting meat
- positioning food items within reach
- occasional assistance initiating a hand-to-mouth pattern
- learning to effectively use adaptive equipment.

The feeding aide's role is important in encouraging maximal independence through verbal assistance rather than unnecessary physical assistance. This group may also need repositioning in wheelchairs, verbal cuing, and physical assistance to get to and from the dining room.

The next level is the **restorative feeding group.** Here, a small group (four to six patients) has one restorative aide to supervise the group and promote the goals established by the occupational therapist. This group eats in a distraction-free area where physical and verbal assistance to complete a meal ranges between maximal assistance and no assistance.

Socially acceptable mealtime behavior and general socializations are reinforced. In order to achieve maximal independence, these patients may require more adaptive equipment as well as monitoring of body position while eating.

The next level is the **dependent feeding group.** This group is for patients who require maximal physical assistance to complete a meal. These patients also require frequent repositioning throughout the meal in order to achieve a good eating posture. These patients are generally not aware of socially acceptable mealtime behavior and are more dependent in functional mobility. One-to-one assistance is needed in order to get adequate nutrition.

The lowest functioning feeding level is the **tube feeding group.** These patients receive nutrition via nasogastric tubes or the various types of gastrostomy tubes. These patients are usually situated in their rooms and are monitored closely by the nursing staff in order to prevent reflux or aspiration. Proper body positioning and oral care are most important for these patients.

Appendix F

Dysphagia-Training Videotapes

A number of dysphagia-training videotapes are commercially available. Here are just a few.

From Communication Skill Builders
3830 E. Bellevue/P.O. Box 42050
Tucson, AZ 85733
(602) 323-7500

> *Managing Dysphagia: An Instructional Guide for the Client and Family* by Brad Hutchins. Includes videotape, clinician's guide, and client handbooks.

From Northern Speech Services, Inc.
117 North Elm Street
P.O. Box 1247
Gaylord, MI 49735
(517) 732-3866

> *Precautions for Feeding Dysphagic Patients: An Inservice Training Program for Feeding Staff.* Includes videotape, in-service manuals, and feeding plan forms.
>
> *The Diagnosis and Treatment of Dysphagia.* Includes slides, manual and videotape.
>
> *Physiological and Anatomic Oropharyngeal Swallowing Disorders.* Includes videotape and manual.

From Mt. Zion Hospital and Medical Center
1600 Divisadero
San Francisco, CA 94115
(415) 567-6600

> *Management of the Dysphagic Patient.*

From Co Productions Australia
103 Fisher St.
Fullarton, South Australia
5063 Australia

> *Dysphagia: A Hard Act to Swallow* by Anita Serradura and Peter Hill. Includes videotape and manual.

From University of Washington Press
P.O. Box 50096
Seattle, WA 98145-5096

> *Dysphagia: How to Feed a Patient Safely* by Susan S. Coombes and Kathy Ware. Includes videotape, instruction manual, and student handbook.

Suppliers of Adaptive Equipment

Adaptive equipment is available from a number of commercial suppliers. Here are just a few.

Smith and Nephew Rolyan, Inc.
Activities of Daily Living Products
N93 W14475 Whittaker Way
Menomonee Falls, WI 53051

(800) 558-8633
(In Wisconsin: 1-800-722-0442)

Enrichments for Better Living
145 Tower Drive
P.O. Box 579
Hinsdale, IL 60521

(800) 323-5547

Flaghouse Rehab
150 N. MacQuesten Pkwy.
Mt. Vernon, NY 10550

(800) 221-5185 or (914) 699-1900

North Coast Medical, Inc.
187 Stauffer Blvd.
San Jose, CA 95125-1042

(800) 821-9319

Fred Sammons, Inc.
Professional Healthcare Catalog
PO Box 32
Brookfield, IL 60513-0032

(800) 323-5547

Sears Health Care
Customer Service Department 731A
Sears Tower
Chicago, IL 60684

(800) 366-3000

Appendix H

Calculating Percentage of Food Intake
Breakfast

MONDAY

	0%	25%	50%	75%	100%
Eggs					
Bacon					
Toast					
Cereal					

Total % ____________

TUESDAY

	0%	25%	50%	75%	100%
Eggs					
Bacon					
Toast					
Cereal					

Total % ____________

WEDNESDAY

	0%	25%	50%	75%	100%
Eggs					
Bacon					
Toast					
Cereal					

Total % ____________

THURSDAY

	0%	25%	50%	75%	100%
Eggs					
Bacon					
Toast					
Cereal					

Total % ____________

FRIDAY

	0%	25%	50%	75%	100%
Eggs					
Bacon					
Toast					
Cereal					

Total % ____________

SATURDAY

	0%	25%	50%	75%	100%
Eggs					
Bacon					
Toast					
Cereal					

Total % ____________

SUNDAY

	0%	25%	50%	75%	100%
Eggs					
Bacon					
Toast					
Cereal					

Total % ____________

SUMMARY

Total % = ______________

7 meals

Average percentage of this meal consumed

Total % = ______________

Calculating Percentage of Food Intake
Lunch

MONDAY

	0%	25%	50%	75%	100%
Meat					
Starch					
Vegetables					
Fruit					
Bread					
Dessert					

Total % _____

TUESDAY

	0%	25%	50%	75%	100%
Meat					
Starch					
Vegetables					
Fruit					
Bread					
Dessert					

Total % _____

WEDNESDAY

	0%	25%	50%	75%	100%
Meat					
Starch					
Vegetables					
Fruit					
Bread					
Dessert					

Total % _____

THURSDAY

	0%	25%	50%	75%	100%
Meat					
Starch					
Vegetables					
Fruit					
Bread					
Dessert					

Total % _____

FRIDAY

	0%	25%	50%	75%	100%
Meat					
Starch					
Vegetables					
Fruit					
Bread					
Dessert					

Total % _____

SATURDAY

	0%	25%	50%	75%	100%
Meat					
Starch					
Vegetables					
Fruit					
Bread					
Dessert					

Total % _____

SUNDAY

	0%	25%	50%	75%	100%
Meat					
Starch					
Vegetables					
Fruit					
Bread					
Dessert					

Total % _____

SUMMARY

Total % = _____

7 meals

Average percentage of this meal consumed

Total % = _____

Calculating Percentage of Food Intake
Dinner

MONDAY

	0%	25%	50%	75%	100%
Meat					
Starch					
Vegetables					
Fruit					
Bread					
Dessert					

Total % _____

TUESDAY

	0%	25%	50%	75%	100%
Meat					
Starch					
Vegetables					
Fruit					
Bread					
Dessert					

Total % _____

WEDNESDAY

	0%	25%	50%	75%	100%
Meat					
Starch					
Vegetables					
Fruit					
Bread					
Dessert					

Total % _____

THURSDAY

	0%	25%	50%	75%	100%
Meat					
Starch					
Vegetables					
Fruit					
Bread					
Dessert					

Total % _____

FRIDAY

	0%	25%	50%	75%	100%
Meat					
Starch					
Vegetables					
Fruit					
Bread					
Dessert					

Total % _____

SATURDAY

	0%	25%	50%	75%	100%
Meat					
Starch					
Vegetables					
Fruit					
Bread					
Dessert					

Total % _____

SUNDAY

	0%	25%	50%	75%	100%
Meat					
Starch					
Vegetables					
Fruit					
Bread					
Dessert					

Total % _____

SUMMARY

Total % = _____

7 meals

Average percentage of this meal consumed

Total % = _____

Calorie Count Record

Food served	Amount consumed	Calories	Protein (grams)
Breakfast			
10:00 AM			
Lunch			
2:00 PM			
Dinner			
H.S.			
TOTALS			

Name_____

Date _____ Room _____

Practical Hints for Preparing Foods at Home

Suggested equipment

food blender or processor

measuring cup

measuring spoons

scale

Recommended daily requirements

Meats—2 or more servings per day (1 serving = 3 oz.)

Milk/milk products—2 or more cups per day

Breads/cereals—4 or more servings per day (1 serving = ½ cup)

Gravy, salad dressings, ice cream, gelatin, soft drinks, coffee, tea, milk shakes

Extra foods may be needed to fulfill caloric needs

Suggestions

☞ Use approximately twice as much food as you normally would for each serving. The caloric intake needs may be higher for your family member. Also, the puree process tends to break food down to a lesser amount.

☞ Make more than one meal at a time. Store surplus in individual serving bowls, frozen for future use.

☞ Remember: taste and appearance are vital. Use your imagination to make food as attractive as possible.

☞ To puree food, add bouillon soups or milk to moisten prepared foods. Place food in blender and use "puree" setting. Add extra liquid as needed.

☞ For mechanical soft diets, use the blender's "chop" setting.

☞ To thicken pureed food, add small amounts of instant potato flakes.

☞ Frozen or fresh cooked vegetables puree more effectively than do canned foods.

☞ Prepare foods your family member has enjoyed in the past.

☞ Small toothbrushes may be used to clean teeth after eating. Flavored swabs or glycerin sticks may be used to clean gums and the oral cavity.

The Quality Assurance Form

Use the *Quality Assurance Form* to record the patient's progress and status regarding feeding, swallowing, and diet consistency while the patient is under the care of the multidisciplinary swallowing team. On page 120 is a sample form; a reproducible blank form is included on page 122.

Completing the Quality Assurance Form

Complete this form at the team meeting when the patient is discharged from the multidisciplinary team program.

1. **Patient initials.** Write patient's initials and hospital or medical record identification number.

2. **Medical diagnosis.** Write medical diagnosis as related to patient's dysphagia.

   Nutritional intake. Note method by which nutrition is received (such as nasogastric tube).

3. **Initial dysphagia diagnosis.** Write diagnosis as determined by speech-language pathology evaluation. If screening only was administered, a diagnosis is not made.

4. **Evaluation date.** Write date of first evaluation by speech-language pathologist and/or other members of team.

5. **ST/OT 1:1 P.O. intake.** Write date when speech-language pathologist and/or occupational therapist first attempted oral feeding after initial evaluation. If patient is feeding by mouth, or if any oral feeding is determined to be unsafe (including trial feeding), write "not applicable" in this space.

6. **Nursing 1:1 P.O. intake.** Same as no. 5, except trained nursing personnel administer oral feeding.

7. **Date to restorative feeding program.** Write date patient advanced to small group, supervised situation.

8. **Date D/C tube feeding.** Write date tube feeding was discontinued.

9. **D/C feeding situation.** Enter method by which nutrition is received, and where. If patient is receiving oral feeding, note whether feeding is in room, small group, large group. Also note amount of supervision or if patient is independent.

10. **D/C diet.** Write consistency of diet at time of patient's discharge from multidisciplinary team.

11. **D/C dysphagia diagnosis.** At time of patient's discharge from team, write dysphagia diagnosis as determined by speech-language pathology.

12. **D/C date.** Write date patient is discharged from multidisciplinary team program.

    Duration. Write number of days from initial evaluation to discharged date.

13. **Comments.** Write therapies received, medical complications, hospitalizations.

Quality Assurance Form

1 Pt. Initials ID#	2 Med. DX Nutritional intake	3 Initial dysphagia DX	4 Evaluation date	5 ST/OT 1:1 P.O. intake	6 Nursing 1:1 P.O. intake	7 Date to restorative feeding program	8 Date D/C Tube feeding	9 D/C Feeding situation	10 D/C Diet	11 D/C Dysphagia DX	12 D/C Date Duration	13 Comments Therapies Complications, etc.
LP 13662	Pneumonia, dementia puree, fed by nursing	Unable to safely feed self 2° dementia	OT 3/9/xx ST screening 3/16/xx	n/a	3/7/xx	n/a	n/a	1:1 nursing assistance in dining room	puree	same	3/16/xx 7 days	nursing to follow
WB 133399	R CVA PEG	mild	re-eval. 3/26/xx videofluoroscopic study 3/21/xx	3/26/xx	4/9/xx	n/a	4/25/xx	Independent feeder, nursing supervision in dining room	puree with mech. soft meat	mild	5/21/xx 56 days	Pt D/C home
LG 113761	Parkinson's Disease Retention Cyst (1) feeder mechanical soft diet	Hx of esophageal 2° retention cyst	3/28/xx	n/a	n/a	n/a	n/a	dining room supervision	mech. soft	resolved	4/4/xx 8 days	ST for voice D/C 4/11/xx
MM 13811	L CVA NG tube	severe non-functional	4/11/xx	n/a	n/a	n/a	n/a	Ng tube	Ng tube	severe non-functional	4/24/xx 14 days	Pt D/C to hospital for PEG placement
LS 113860	CA of colon; post-op hemicolectomy; mult. intubations regular diet self-feeder	mild	5/3/xx 5/4/xx	n/a	n/a	n/a	n/a	self-feeder in room	puree	mild	5/23/xx 20 days	PT, OT, ST D/C home

Quality Assurance Form: Summary of Sample Entries

Dates included: 3-90 through 5-90 (3 months)

Number of patients: 5

Number of patients receiving non-oral feedings on admission to team program: 2

Number of patients receiving non-oral feedings on discharge from team program: 1

Number of patients with the following dysphagia diagnoses

	Initially	*Discharge*
Severe, nonfunctional	2	2
Moderately severe		
Moderate		
Mild-moderate	1	
Mild	2	2
Minimal		
Normal		1

Average duration: 21.0 days

Number of patients with aspiration pneumonia

Initially	*Discharge*
1	1

Number of patients requiring changes in diet consistency: 3

Quality Assurance Form

1	2	3	4	5	6	7	8	9	10	11	12	13
Pt. Initials ID#	Med. DX Nutritional intake	Initial dysphagia DX	Evaluation date	ST/OT 1:1 P.O. intake	Nursing 1:1 P.O. intake	Date to restorative feeding program	Date D/C Tube feeding	D/C Feeding situation	D/C Diet	D/C Dysphagia DX	D/C Date Duration	Comments Therapies Complications, etc.